W9-DIU-188

Caring and Community

Concepts and Models
for Service-Learning
in **Nursing**

Jane S. Norbeck, Charlene Connolly, and JoEllen Koerner, volume editors

Edward Zlotkowski, series editor

A PUBLICATION OF THE

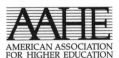

AMERICAN ASSOCIATION
FOR HIGHER EDUCATION

Published in cooperation with Community-Campus Partnerships for Health

Acknowledgments

The editors express deep appreciation to Ms. Barbara Mow for her masterful organizational and communication skills that kept all contributors informed and on target. Her work in attending to the details of format and style resulted in a unified monograph. Without her careful follow-up over the course of many months, this project would not have been completed on schedule or with the quality that resulted.

This monograph was published in cooperation with:

Community-Campus Partnerships for Health
1388 Sutter Street, Suite 805
San Francisco, CA 94109
ph 415/502-7979, fax 415/476-4113
email ccph@itsa.ucsf.edu
http://futurehealth.ucsf.edu

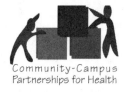

Community-Campus
Partnerships for Health

Caring and Community: Concepts and Models for Service-Learning in Nursing
(AAHE's Series on Service-Learning in the Disciplines)
Jane S. Norbeck, Charlene Connolly, and JoEllen Koerner, *volume editors*
Edward Zlotkowski, *series editor*

ISBN 1-56377-009-1
ISBN (18 vol. set) 1-56377-005-9

Contents

Samples of Syllabi and Assignments

Appendix

About This Series

by Edward Zlotkowski

The following volume, *Caring and Community: Concepts and Models for Service-Learning in Nursing*, represents the fourth in a series of monographs on service-learning and the academic disciplines. Ever since the early 1990s, educators interested in reconnecting higher education not only with neighboring communities but also with the American tradition of education for service have recognized the critical importance of winning faculty support for this work. Faculty, however, tend to define themselves and their responsibilities largely in terms of the academic disciplines/interdisciplinary areas in which they have been trained. Hence, the logic of the present series.

The idea for this series first surfaced approximately three years ago at a meeting convened by Campus Compact to explore the feasibility of developing a national network of service-learning educators. At that meeting, it quickly became clear that some of those assembled saw the primary value of such a network in its ability to provide concrete resources to faculty working in or wishing to explore service-learning. Out of that meeting there developed, under the auspices of Campus Compact, a new national group of educators called the Invisible College, and it was within the Invisible College that the monograph project was first conceived. Indeed, a review of both the editors and contributors responsible for many of the volumes in this series would reveal significant representation by faculty associated with the Invisible College.

If Campus Compact helped supply the initial financial backing and impulse for the Invisible College and for this series, it was the American Association for Higher Education (AAHE) that made completion of the project feasible. Thanks to its reputation for innovative work, AAHE was not only able to obtain the funding needed to support the project up through actual publication, it was also able to assist in attracting many of the teacher-scholars who participated as writers and editors.

Three individuals in particular deserve to be singled out for their contributions. Sandra Enos, former Campus Compact project director for Integrating Service and Academic Study, was shepherd to the Invisible College project. John Wallace, professor of philosophy at the University of Minnesota, was the driving force behind the creation of the Invisible College. Without his vision and faith in the possibility of such an undertaking, assembling the human resources needed for this series would have been very difficult. Third, AAHE's endorsement — and all that followed in its wake — was due largely to AAHE vice president Lou Albert. Lou's enthusiasm for

the monograph project and his determination to see it adequately supported have been critical to its success. It is to Sandra, John, and Lou that the
monograph series as a whole must be dedicated.

Other individuals to whom the series owes a special note of thanks
include Matt Bliss, who, as my graduate assistant, helped set up many of the
communications mechanisms that got the project started, and Jeannette
MacInnes, coordinator of student programs at the Bentley Service-Learning
Center, who has served as a reliable source of both practical and moral
support.

The Rationale Behind the Series

A few words should be said at this point about the makeup of both the general series and the individual volumes. Although nursing may seem a natural choice of disciplines with which to link service-learning, given nursing's
intrinsic relationship to service, "natural fit" has not, in fact, been a deter-
minant factor in deciding which disciplines/interdisciplinary areas the
series should include. Far more important have been considerations related
to the overall range of disciplines represented. Since experience has shown
that there is probably no disciplinary area — from architecture to zoology —
where service-learning cannot be fruitfully employed to strengthen students' abilities to become active learners as well as responsible citizens, a
primary goal in putting the series together has been to demonstrate this
fact. Thus, some rather natural choices for inclusion — disciplines such as
anthropology, geography, and religious studies — have been passed over in
favor of other, sometimes less obvious selections from the business disciplines and natural sciences as well as several important interdisciplinary
areas. Should the present series of volumes prove useful and well received,
we can then consider filling in the many gaps we have left this first time
around.

If a concern for variety has helped shape the series as a whole, a concern for legitimacy has been central to the design of the individual volumes.
To this end, each volume has been both written by and aimed primarily at
academics working in a particular disciplinary/interdisciplinary area. Many
individual volumes have, in fact, been produced with the encouragement
and active support of relevant discipline-specific national societies. For this
volume, in fact, we owe thanks to the Community-Campus Partnerships for
Health.

Furthermore, each volume has been designed to include its own appropriate theoretical, pedagogical, and bibliographical material. Especially with
regard to theoretical and bibliographical material, this design has resulted in
considerable variation both in quantity and in level of discourse. Thus, for

example, a volume such as Accounting contains more introductory and less bibliographical material than does Composition — simply because there is less written on and less familiarity with service-learning in accounting. However, no volume is meant to provide an extended introduction to service-learning *as a generic concept*. For material of this nature, the reader is referred to such texts as Kendall's *Combining Service and Learning: A Resource Book for Community and Public Service* (NSIEE, 1990) and Jacoby's *Service-Learning in Higher Education* (Jossey-Bass, 1996).

I would like to conclude with a note of special thanks to Jane Norbeck, Charlene Connolly, and JoEllen Koerner, coeditors of the Nursing monograph. Rarely have I had the pleasure of working with colleagues whose academic expertise has been complemented by such a remarkable attention to punctuality and procedural details. I would also like to acknowledge the generous assistance of Julie Sebastian of the University of Kentucky, who provided valuable feedback on the manuscript.

October 1997

Introduction

by Jane S. Norbeck, Charlene Connolly, and JoEllen Koerner

Envisioning a monograph series on service-learning in nursing would, at first thought, yield chapters with expected, predictable outcomes. After all, nursing has historically been and continues to be a provider of service and an advocate for quality care. In addition, nursing has sought to promote individual health, extending as well to communities.

But nursing as a profession within academic, research, and health-care organizations has not, until recently, begun to embrace true service-learning. The chapters in this monograph are rich with information, both theoretical and experiential, that describes ways in which nursing has begun to incorporate service-learning as a methodology into many diverse settings and with communities of interest.

Although there are many definitions of service-learning, basic elements of similarity emerge that are integral to the foundation of service-learning. Service-learning is an instructional methodology built upon a foundation of experiential learning enhanced by critical, reflective thinking. Through community service, participants have opportunities to enhance their civic and social responsibilities and to develop critical-thinking and group problem-solving competencies.

The National and Community Service Trust Act of 1993 defines service-learning as:

> . . . *a method under which students or participants learn and develop through active participation in thoughtfully organized service that is conducted in and meets the needs of a community and is coordinated with an elementary school, secondary school, institution of higher education, or community-service program, and with the community, helps foster civic and social responsibility, is integrated into and enhances the academic curriculum of the student's program or the educational competencies of the community-service program in which the participants are enrolled, and includes structured time for the students and participants to reflect on the service experience.*

The Corporation for National Service has defined two core elements as essential to service-learning: (1) Service activities help meet community needs that *the community* identifies as important, and (2) educational components are structured to enhance critical thinking and reflection on the service activities and community needs.

Service-learning not only connects theory with application and practice but also creates an environment where both the provider of service and the recipient learn from each other. Although essentially associated with pedagogy and curricular revision, service-learning engages participants in opportunities to explore the civic and social responsibilities of nursing education, practice, and research perspectives.

The provider sector of health care has also recognized the value of and opportunities for change through service-learning. As isolated hospital and agency care moves toward integrated systems with a focus on healthy communities, a natural environment and structure for shared learning and development emerges. Several health systems have used innovative service-learning approaches to join with consumers in identifying issues for health service agendas. Others have created new relationships between the service agencies and medical, nursing, and allied health students in teaching-learning models that actively involve clients in codesigning plans of care. Interdependence in education and service is replacing the narrow and often costly autonomous models of the past.

From the research perspective, service-learning provides rich opportunities. Evaluation research is needed at two levels: evaluation of student learning and development, and evaluation of the outcomes of the service delivery at the community level. Multivariate theory testing studies need to be designed to test relationships among student characteristics, characteristics of service-learning projects, and selected types of learning and service outcomes.

Substantive Issues Raised by the Chapters

Through their experiences in service-learning, the contributing authors have raised issues that continue to need dialogue and resolution. Some questions that have surfaced are these: how to create meaningful connections beyond the requirements of patient care, how to coalesce fragmented nursing curricula, and how to develop a central focus on the individual in the context of the community as health care shifts to that setting. An ethical issue involves recognizing the resources and strengths that consumers and communities bring to a relationship and ensuring that service-learning is not embraced and implemented at the expense of the community.

The change that is required to engage in service-learning has emerged as challenges to nurses at many levels. Some faculty erroneously believe that through the service they provide they are already engaged in service-learning. Acute-care nurses need to be empowered themselves to provide care in community-based settings while simultaneously assisting the community to become more empowered. As health-care organizations are introducing academic content related to organizational change through service-learning, they are challenged to build community and transform their organizations into learning organizations.

The need for careful mentoring and support for students as they undergo changes in the learning process has been noted. Developing critical-thinking concepts, refocusing on civic and social responsibilities for healthy communities, identifying community resources, and noting the causative agents impeding the health of communities are new paradigms of learning for all levels of nursing students.

Broad implications affecting faculty, students, the community, and the curriculum have been found in relation to the shift in clinical settings toward community-based care. The need for faculty to develop more skills and greater flexibility when coordinating service-learning experiences involves acknowledging themselves as learners as well as educators and providers of service. In a broader sense, concerns have been identified regarding the relationship between nursing educators and providers as the large nationally funded programs aimed at restructuring the health-care delivery system have been implemented.

Along with these and other substantive issues, the strength of this monograph lies in the richness of experience nursing is able to bring to the changing dynamics of the health-care industry as well as the complexities of our communities as we enter a new century.

Key Concepts

Several concepts, key to nursing practice, make up the framework for this document. However, they are expressed with an enlarged definition, demonstrating the continuing adaptation of nursing to a changing and complex world.

Community is a major theme in many chapters. The nursing discipline has long viewed community as a specific group, bound together by shared interests, needs, and values. Community is now being conceptualized as a process, a convening and converging of loosely coupled groups for a specific purpose or period. Nursing, the catalyst for this assemblage of persons, provides a focus on quality of life that transcends the narrower frame of disease management.

The notion of *academia* as the site for teaching and clinical institutions has also been expanded. The clear line of demarcation is softening as academic settings establish clinical-care services and health-care settings instill a teaching-learning philosophy. A deeper shift in focus is noted when a whole community becomes a primary site both for teaching and for service. This model views each person as expert on his/her own life and worldview, capitalizing on the richness of shared perspectives to create an inter-dependence and interrelationship based on mutuality and shared under-standing.

Finally, the foundational notion of *health*, the focus of professional nurs-ing, has been enlarged. Following the models of modern physics, the 1970s and 1980s behavioral psychosocial definition of health focused on a balance among body-mind-spirit through adaptation. The radical discoveries of post-modern physics provide a more contemporary view of health based on a sci-ence of living systems. In this view, health is defined as a balance between the individual and the environment, an expansion of consciousness/ awareness that increases choices, and the process of living the values one chooses. In each of these definitions of health, the focus is extended beyond the individual to include his or her relationships with the external world of people and things. In this model, the person is expert on his or her life and what constitutes health, not the health-care provider. The role of nursing is to serve as a catalyst to facilitate choices that lead to enriched patterns of living.

Thus, the book is a story of partnerships between education and service, between nurse and person, between profession and community. This rich network of interrelationships focused on biological, physical, social, cultur-al, and spiritual phenomena creates a sustaining web of life for a public we are privileged to serve.

Plan of the Monograph

The monograph opens with a chapter that connects humanistic learning with professional development and describes how service-learning provides opportunities for extending professional education into the realm of devel-oping capacity for dealing with values and judgment. The next two chapters in Part 1 give an aerial view of the scope of service-learning projects that have emerged in nursing. The first describes two foundation-funded initia-tives in nursing that provided opportunities for projects across the nation to focus on service-learning in the context of improving nursing services or enhancing opportunities for nursing education. The second aerial view depicts an impressive range of services and funding sources made possible through the work of a consortium that developed service-learning experi-ences as an outgrowth of its search for new models of effective health care. These service-learning initiatives served as a catalyst to the discovery of community needs and ways to meet them.

Part 2 shifts gears: Here the chapter authors provide descriptions of spe-cific service-learning programs and experiences and share insights on prac-tical issues involved in planning and implementing service-learning in the curriculum. A common theme across these seven case-study chapters is the emphasis on underserved and vulnerable groups: elderly, poor, uninsured, immigrant — all populations with needs that transcend traditional medically focused care. The chapters in this section are presented according to increasing interdisciplinary complexity or inclusiveness of the student participants. "Service-Learning as a Pedagogy" describes service-learning opportunities for baccalaureate nursing students through a variety of community projects focused on health, such as diabetic screening or hospice care. "Case Study of a Service-Learning Project in a Nurse-Managed Clinic" describes a community health nursing practicum focused on primary care for homeless and indigent individuals that was developed in conjunction with a campuswide service-learning course. "A Case Study in Service-Learning Using a Collaborative Community-Based Caring Model" introduces a modified differentiated practice model to guide the inclusion of nursing students from three levels (associate's, baccalaureate, and master's) along with allied health students, and presents a case study to illustrate the roles for these levels and disciplines. The interdisciplinary mix is further expanded in "Community Empowerment," which describes a community empowerment project that included graduate students from nursing, medicine, and social work. Undergraduate nursing students in pediatric or community health courses participated with students from the departments of social work, medicine, professional psychology, dental hygiene, and dietetic technology in projects to improve child health in an urban public school ("Nursing Clinical Education"). "The Community as Classroom" describes an even more comprehensive team-based approach that included students from nursing, medicine, occupational therapy, physical therapy, hearing and speech pathology, nutrition, environmental health, and health education, who worked to improve the health status of an isolated rural community. The final chapter in this section ("Service-Learning Lessons") takes us the farthest afield but also shows us how some of the ideas already embodied in more familiar settings can be extended beyond the academy proper. Practical as the case study chapters are, they also provide interesting insights as well as clear accounts of strategies to facilitate the development of critical thinking and reflection on service activities and community needs.

The rest of the monograph offers even more specific tools for people interested in developing service-learning: sample course materials, including syllabi, assignments, and student projects; an annotated bibliography; and a list of resource persons.

Several of the chapter authors spontaneously provided historical context describing linkages between aspects of service-learning and the historical roots and traditions of nursing. The first essay chapter notes that humanistic learning has been foundational to collegiate nursing education since 1893, and two of the case study chapters trace the historical linkages with service in nursing. Yet service-learning includes additional elements beyond those traditionally found in the service orientation of nursing education. These elements have been incorporated into the programs described in the monograph, resulting in exciting new dimensions in the formative experiences of nurses that should prepare them for leadership roles in the health-care systems of the future. Through embracing service-learning and community, nursing curricula have been expanded and enriched — thus our title: "Caring and Community."

Humanistic Learning in the Context of Service:
The Liberal Arts in Nursing Education

by Jean E. Bartels

The Place of Humanistic Learning in College Missions

Walk through any college or university campus and you will most likely find, etched into the very stone and wood of the buildings, the promises of higher education: Truth, Character, Justice, Liberty, Understanding, Honesty, Courage, Wisdom, Enlightenment, Beauty. In these times of growing debate over the purposes of higher education, there remains clear agreement that the academic experience should aim to prepare students to assume their roles as good stewards of the human endeavor.

To use the 2,000-year-old words of Plato from *The Republic,* "If you ask what is the good of education, the answer is easy — that education makes good [people] and that good [people] act nobly." Mission statements of colleges and universities consistently speak to the development of students as responsible citizens, prepared to provide leadership through service to society. Academic preparation brings with it the obligation for graduates to think, act, and serve as responsible citizens. It is through humanistic liberal education that students learn to enter the intellectual debate, explore the origins and destiny of the human enterprise, understand and challenge the values, ethics, and mores of civilization, and begin to hone the skills of relationship building. It is through service-learning, however, that students begin to understand and practice their roles as responsible trustees of the human community.

The philosophy and meaning of a liberal education provide a powerful underpinning for understanding the place of service and citizenship in the development of professionals. It is the purpose of this chapter to connect humanistic liberal learning with professional development through the opportunities of service-learning.

The Focus of Humanistic Learning for the Professions

As we enter the 21st century, the debates over the purposes of a humanistic liberal arts education have intensified to almost crisis proportions. While once a liberal education was thought to be essential for the development of a group of elite individuals destined for positions of authority in the governing class, it has since come to be the privilege of the many who enter the higher academic community. Within today's context, most believe that a liberal education prepares all educated individuals with the skills and abilities necessary for active participation in both shaping and leading a democratic society. As such, a humanistic education encourages creative thinking that not only welcomes but actively seeks diverse perspectives, thus stimulating a larger worldview.

By contrast, some argue that the role of higher academia should be to prepare workers for professions and careers. Within this context, a liberal education, it is believed, should be narrowed or restricted to allow important time for the transfer of significant information and workplace skills related to a useful trade. Most would agree, however, that these very professionals should be characterized by their ability to link their knowledge with appropriate values and judgments when making complex decisions in their field. Without a solid base in liberal studies and humanistic learning experiences, these professional attributes can hardly be realized.

Giroux and Kaye (1989) argue that "today's crisis in liberal education is one of historical purpose and meaning, a crisis that challenges us to rethink the most fundamental relationships between the role of the university and the imperatives of democracy in a mass society" (A44). These authors advocate for the education of a critical citizen — a professional who has experienced the connection of both liberal education and career preparation. Humanistic learning and professional studies can combine to support the development of thoughtful, active citizens. In fact, they must if we are to avoid artificial distinctions between education for life and education for work.

The essence of a liberal education goes beyond the development of career-specific skills to the development of values and approaches needed to resolve the experiences of life. A complete education allows students both to understand themselves and to act with the conviction of their perspectives. Done well, a humanistic, liberal education fosters:

Perspective — *the awareness that the way things are is not the way they always have been or the way they must necessarily be in the future*
Critique — *the deliberate ability to unveil and dereify existing canon and dogma in order to comprehend and reveal the social origins of the political, economic, and cultural orders in which we live and have lived*
Consciousness — *the appreciation of the making of history*
Remembrance — *the ability to acknowledge the past as a reservoir of experience — both tragic and hopeful — from which we draw in order to act*
Imagination — *the recognition of the present as history, thus enabling the consideration of the structures, movement, and possibilities of a contempo-*

rary world as a laboratory to show us how we might act to prevent the bar-baric and develop the humanistic. (Giroux and Kaye 1989: A44)

It is from these perspectives that a clear definition of humanistic liberal education can be drawn and a context for the role of service-learning in nursing education can be defined.

Toward a Definition of Humanistic Learning for the Professions

The literature is replete with definitions of humanistic learning in higher education. Humanistic learning, a blending of the liberal arts and sciences, "offers a deep breath, a broad vision, filled with the buzzing confusion and glory of human possibility. Oriented toward the development of individual judgment, such learning provides the intellectual independence and empathic understanding that are the foundation of democracy" (Grumet 1995: 4). A liberal education implies the formation of habits of free inquiry, of reflection, of an unprejudiced search for the truth, and of a deliberately chosen responsibility for doing social good.

It is the goal of a liberal education to cultivate the critical-thinking abilities of students, to liberate their minds so that they might pursue a lifelong search for understanding and truth, and to stimulate their thoughtful reflection and action (Eisenhauer and O'Neil 1995: 12). Educators in every discipline and profession hope, somehow, to prepare graduates who can recognize the profound complexity of questions facing their practice, who can appreciate the moral, ethical, and practical impact of the judgments they must make, and who can thoughtfully and sensitively act with honesty, courage, and flexibility (Read 1980). These expectations can be met only when education provides connected opportunities for faculty and students alike to immerse themselves in the active work of applied learning. In fact, learning is incomplete unless students have the opportunity to test their learning in service to others, reflecting on the strengths and weaknesses of their personal contributions.

Humanistic Learning in the Context of Nursing Education

A comprehensive review of nursing literature from 1893 to 1939 completed by Hanson (1989, 1991) demonstrates that the expectations for humanistic learning have long been foundational to college- and university-based nursing education. Nurse educators have consistently believed that a liberal education contributes both the intellectual skills and cognitive knowledge base required for nursing practice. It encourages the development of the individual, provides for the acquisition of knowledge in the sciences and humanities, promotes cultural competence, develops needed critical-thinking skills, and prepares graduates for roles as effective citizens and leaders in social reform initiatives.

Nurse educators today concur but also recognize that rapid, unpredictable changes in health care will additionally require that graduates can analyze, synthesize, and act wisely, ethically, and with accountability on behalf of their patients (Eisenhauer and O'Neil 1995). It is in the application of these foundational arts that professional nurses learn the clinical judgment skills required for practice in traditional clinical practica. However, it is in the experience of providing service that they gain the personal insights required for them to act on behalf of those experiencing social injustice and learn their role as guardians and servants of the community. It is in the study of the profession that the students of nursing learn to focus their expertise. It is in the delivery of service that they earn the sanction that permits them to act with responsibility in the world. Nursing's social contract obliges students to assume the obligation and privilege of intervening in other people's lives, their learning, health, and worldly affairs. As professionals, they are to develop the ethics and discipline their practice requires. Their entire education is aimed toward service to society (Grumet 1995).

The American Association of Colleges of Nursing, in its *Essentials of College and University Education for Professional Nursing* (1986), also recognizes that graduates of professional nursing programs must develop the "qualities of mind and character that are necessary to live a free and fulfilling life, act in the public interest locally and globally, and contribute to health-care improvements and the nursing profession" (7). These attributes require focused experiences beyond the classroom and traditional clinical practica. If learning is to be effective, producing a reflective, socially engaged practitioner, it needs to be housed in the context of service experiences developed over time.

The Liberal Arts as a Cornerstone in Developing Professional Citizenship

Within the context of both liberal learning and nursing education, it is clear that there is an expectation that students develop a sense of responsibility as citizens of a democratic society. A democratic society requires a citizenry who are able to think clearly and critically on issues, to understand the interdependent nature of social existence, to appreciate the diversity of values and the aesthetic of difference, to judge with a spirit of compassion, and to problem solve effectively for the good of the whole. It is the very nature of humanistic, liberal education that these abilities be developed.

The arts and humanities give voice to the history, values, experiences, and aesthetics of diverse peoples. They provide a vision of how communities and societies are shaped and sustained, how they creatively express themselves and flourish across time and cultures. The behavioral and social sciences afford a window to view how individuals and groups experience and adjust to divergent expectations in multiple cultural contexts. They examine the ebb and flow of individual development and the function of human systems. The natural and mathematical sciences explore and expand the boundaries of the material world, stretching the human capacity to reason, solve problems, investigate, and construct reality.

These bodies of knowledge and academic abilities mean little, however, if they are not tested in engagement with the social community. Education for democracy means education for participation in an increasingly diverse world. It requires immersion in multiple perspectives and reflection on multiple, diverse interactions and involvements. As Battistoni (1995) advises, what is needed is the "integration of liberal teaching, experiential learning, critical reflection, community service, and citizen education into a pedagogy of freedom" (35). Service-learning provides the needed linkage for such expectations. As defined in this volume's introduction, "Service-learning is . . . built upon a foundation of experiential learning enhanced by critical, reflective thinking. Through community service, participants have opportunities to enhance their civic and social responsibilities and to develop critical-thinking and group problem-solving competencies" [see p. 1].

The Abilities of an Effective Professional Citizen

Academic institutions in our country do a magnificent job of preparing professionals with the knowledge of their crafts, the cognitive information that makes them world-class leaders in knowledge generation. Professionals seldom find themselves in difficulty because they have too little information or access to it. They more likely find themselves in trouble because they have not learned to develop the affective, kinesthetic, moral/ethical, and communicative dimensions of their personalities and professional selves. Most students experience education — even quite fine humanistic liberal education — as an isolated set of content capsules that do not promote the development of abilities needed by an integrated professional or a contributing citizen. The Corporation for National Service notes that two core elements must be present for learning to be of service to both the learner and society: Service activities must help meet the needs that the community identifies as important, and educational experiences must be structured to enhance critical thinking and reflection on service activities and community needs.

Alverno College, a liberal arts college for women located in Wisconsin, provides an exemplar of how the integration of liberal arts, professional education, and service-learning can serve both the learner and society. Through the development of eight abilities believed to be necessary for the development of an educated professional, all students at the college experience the integration of professional abilities within the context of their professional and liberal arts education. Building increasing levels of complexity and using content as a context, each course in the curriculum (e.g., all liberal arts, professional studies, and support-area courses) integrates and develops one or more of the abilities necessary for professional development. Regardless of the discipline, all faculty have agreed on the meanings and levels of development of each ability and consistently teach them from a collective perspective. All eight abilities must be mastered at faculty-prescribed levels prior to graduation, many of the eight at advanced levels. Students must develop abilities that will help them put knowledge into action for the rest of their lives:

> **Communication:** *The ability to make connections between self and audience; to speak and write effectively, read and listen critically, use graphics, electronic media, computers, and mathematics to communicate effective messages.*
> **Analysis:** *The ability to think clearly and critically; to fuse experience, reason, and training into considered judgment.*
> **Problem Solving:** *The ability to figure out what the problem is; to find answers that work in different situations; and to get done what needs to be done.*
> **Valuing in Decision Making:** *The ability to recognize different value systems while holding strongly to one's own ethic; to recognize the moral dimensions of decisions and accept responsibility for one's own actions.*
> **Social Interaction:** *The ability to learn how to get things done in committees, task forces, team projects, and other group efforts; to elicit the views of others and help reach conclusions.*
> **Responsibility for the Global Environment:** *The ability to act with an understanding of and respect for the economic, social, and biological interdependence of global life.*
> **Effective Citizenship:** *The development of leadership abilities; to be involved and responsible; to act with an informed awareness of contemporary issues and their historical context.*
> **Aesthetic Responsiveness:** *The ability to understand that some truths are best expressed through the written and performed arts; to appreciate the various forms of art and respond to their symbolism and message.* (paraphrase, Alverno College Faculty 1992: 11-50)

Mastery of these professional, liberal education abilities is accomplished through students' involvement in their learning. What matters is not just what students know, but what they can do with what they know. Learning must be active. While students test out their abilities in traditional clinical experiences and are held responsible for development and self-reflection in experiential classrooms, they also engage in community-based off-campus experiential learning experiences and elective service projects. In each instance, they learn to apply, test out, and refine what they have learned in other courses. They learn to work cooperatively with community members in settings as diverse as shelters for battered women, the Milwaukee AIDS Project, large local corporations and businesses, and central-city free health clinics. While they explore how their studies and abilities go beyond the classroom and across contexts, they also learn how to execute their responsibility as educated persons in service to the expressed needs of their community (Alverno College Faculty 1992, 1994; Alverno College Nursing Faculty 1996).

Integrating Liberal Arts, Professional Studies, and Service-Learning: Developing Connectedness

In far too many instances in higher education, students fail to experience the growth and connectedness that mark optimal progression to professional responsibility. Curricula are often fragmented, independent, disjointed collections of courses where the mastery of content and competition, not the development of the individual, are the central focus. We are in a time when building relationships and recognizing our interdependence across disciplines make such an educational experience not only obsolete but dangerous.

Boyer (1989) admonishes that conceivably "we are educating our students to see themselves in isolation while failing to help them discover their connections; we are stressing their independence but not affirming the interdependent nature of our existence" (102). Take, for example, the following studies, which indicate that nursing students achieve their academic professional goals but fail to involve themselves in activities that would enhance the thinking, action, and service goals of a liberal humanistic education or to see those goals as exceptionally important.

Zaborowska (1995) determined that baccalaureate nursing students placed significant energy into their involvement with academic activities directly associated with their nursing coursework and professional learning. They were less likely, however, to participate in activities that required interaction and engagement with those outside their area of academic study. While students gauged their personal and social development to be high in terms of their ability to understand themselves and others from a values perspective, they failed to recognize how their liberal arts learning impacted their ability to analyze and take multiple perspectives. Although it was clear that students viewed interaction and interpersonal factors as significant contributors to their personal development, much of their education was contained and narrowly defined within the context of their major. Similarly, students did not articulate a sense that their liberal learning experiences prepared them for roles as effective professional citizens.

Equally striking are students' perceptions of their nursing faculty's role in assisting them to clearly link the significance of their liberal arts learning with their professional development and responsibilities. Peck and Jennings (1989) found that, while students believed they made connections between liberal arts and nursing studies, they did so independently. Students made sense of and serendipitously integrated their education by reading texts and discussing their beliefs with other nursing students. Faculty were not identified as factors in assisting them to make links between their educational experiences and requirements for professional involvement and development. Students viewed their clinical practice environments and peers as helpful in broadening their perspectives about their roles as professionals but did not identify any broader connection between their academic learning and the expectation for professional involvement to the broader community. Given these findings, the implications for curriculum development are intriguing.

Creating Integrated, Connected Curricula

Most educators share the assumption that good educators and good curricula naturally develop students' understanding of their roles and responsibilities as professional citizens. However, *better* educators and curricula make the demands of professional citizenship explicit and the linkages between learning experiences and service clear. As educators, we need to look beyond isolated learning experiences to uncover the occurrence and quality of professional development necessary for today's graduates in nursing and, subsequently, connect our expectations to more meaningful, engaging learning experiences. This means creating and reinforcing learning environments that involve students in making actions out of their knowledge — insisting that they use their knowledge in acts of application, generalization, and experimentation in contexts beyond their courses. Such reengineering of our approach to teaching, learning, and curricular development begins quite simply with talking to others.

Through dialogue, we can set forth our collective expectations across courses, programs of nursing study, and the entire college community of learning in order to provide a consistent and public set of demands for student learning and development. By engaging in multidisciplinary inquiry and planned communication across the college faculty, we can isolate a common understanding of our collective expectations for how an educated professional should contribute to society.

Professional citizenship is not developed in a single class taught by a master of humanistic theory or ethics. Such development requires educators to take collective responsibility for teaching, reinforcing, and evaluating each individual student's progress toward meeting the goals clearly articulated in mission and philosophy statements of the program and institution. It requires a common, agreed-upon language and set of developmentally appropriate expectations that students confront in every class they take and from every educator they encounter. It requires an expectation that students are actively engaged in the learning process, are held accountable for carrying learning from one context to another, and are required to make public their commitment to assuming the responsibilities of a professional person through engagement beyond their immediate nursing coursework.

A clear set of publicly articulated outcomes that meet the demands of contemporary society, a planned collection of personally meaningful required service experiences, and a consistent process for ongoing, interdisciplinary feedback to the student can provide a framework for students to question, discover, and reflect on their personal development. Such learning empowers students to move beyond the confines of the classroom and narrow clinical experiences to enter a broader inquiry related to humanistic values and shared social concerns. With consistent faculty guidance and bridging, students can come to recognize how to use a variety of disciplinary frameworks and strategies in analyzing diverse perspectives, how to think and act responsibly with regard to personal and professional concerns, and how to take action with a consistent and informed awareness of contemporary issues.

Boyer (1989) proposes a set of educational strategies that can help us begin to build stronger connections between knowledge and action for ourselves and our students. These suggestions provide a starting point for discussions on teaching-learning expectations between faculty both within and outside our programs. Boyer suggests that we:

> 1. *Grow in students the capacity for clear communication and attention to the quality and integrity of the messages they send. Students should be able to write carefully, think critically, listen with discernment, and speak with power and precision if they are to be personally and socially empowered and connected.* (paraphrase, 104)

What is our common agreement on what clear communication entails? How do we emphasize, analyze, and provide feedback to students regarding their communication styles and abilities as they engage in their developing professional practice? How do we help students recognize the power of their communication in working with and influencing others?

2. Teach students that truth is an obligation they assume when they are empowered by education. Quality is found not only in the content or correctness of our messages but in the integrity of the meanings we share. (104)

What responsibilities do we expect students in our disciplines to assume after graduation? How do we give them experience in recognizing and practicing these responsibilities in their program of studies?

3. Ensure that students learn to put their work into the larger context. Wise professionals cannot work in isolation when our world is increasingly interdependent, socially and ecologically. (104)

How do students demonstrate their ability to envision their professional responsibilities beyond their immediate course experiences? How do we help them see the context of their practice beyond their responsibilities to a "job"?

4. Challenge students to bring moral and ethical perspectives into their professional work. The values professionals bring to their work are every bit as important as the work itself. (104-105)

How do we assure that students have assumed the values of our discipline? How do we test their ability to apply those values in practice?

5. Build collaboration and cooperation into learning environments. Students, as they continue to learn, must accept an obligation to be increasingly engaged in shared responsibility for the serious interdisciplinary problems we face. (106)

How do we move students from a sense of competitive isolation in the academic setting to an understanding of and effectiveness with collaborative inquiry and action? How do we help them to envision their connectedness to others both within and outside their own discipline? Where have we built experiences that force students from their comfortable, isolated learning experiences?

6. Establish the authenticity of connections between the theories of the classroom and the realities of life. Students need to learn how they fit into the larger world. They should understand that the tragedy of life is not death; it is to die with commitments undefined, convictions undeclared, and service unfulfilled. (106-107)

Where and how do our students develop their sense of connectedness to the concerns and issues facing both the professions and society? How do we help them bridge their academic learning into action and commitment? With whom have we built our own learning coalitions as educators?

Obviously, the answers to these questions are complex, and solutions to them present new challenges to our teaching scholarship, our vision of ourselves as educators, and our curricula. What is clear, however, is that none of the questions will be answered without a commitment to a dialogue with others across our own educational and community settings and to the riskful business of expanding the arena of student and faculty learning experiences.

Learning moments outside the classroom and academic teaching environment, those done in service to the wider community, have great potential to allow students to experience a cultural richness beyond that found in any textbook. Ultimately, after all, it will be the humanistic liberal education abilities they possess that will define them as professionals. Best that those abilities be developed in a context grounded in diversity, community, democracy, and public service.

References

Alverno College Faculty. (1992). *Liberal Learning at Alverno College*. Rev. ed. Milwaukee, WI: Alverno Productions.

———. (1994). *Student Assessment-as-Learning at Alverno College*. Rev. ed. Milwaukee, WI: Alverno Productions.

Alverno College Nursing Faculty. (1996). *Nursing Education for the Future: An Outcomes Approach to Teaching, Learning, and Assessment at Alverno College*. Milwaukee, WI: Alverno Productions.

American Association of Colleges of Nursing. (1986). *Essentials of College and University Education for Professional Nursing*. Washington, DC: American Association of Colleges of Nursing.

Battistoni, R. (1995). "Service Learning, Diversity, and the Liberal Arts Curriculum." *Liberal Education* 81(1): 30-35.

Boyer, E. (March/April 1989). "Connectedness Through Liberal Education." *Journal of Professional Nursing* 5(2): 102-107.

Eisenhauer, L., and J. O'Neil. (1995). "Synthesis and Praxis: Liberal Education and Nursing." *Liberal Education* 81(1): 12-17.

Giroux, H., and H. Kaye. (March 29, 1989). "The Liberal Arts Must Be Reformed to Serve Democratic Ends." *Chronicle of Higher Education*: A44.

Grumet, M. (1995). "Lofty Actions and Practical Thoughts: Education With a Purpose." *Liberal Learning* 81(1): 4-9.

Hanson, K. (March/April 1989). "The Emergence of Liberal Education in Nursing Education, 1893-1923." *Journal of Professional Nursing* 5(2): 83-91.

————. (November/December 1991). "An Analysis of the Historical Context of Liberal Education in Nursing Education From 1924 to 1939." *Journal of Professional Nursing* 7(6): 341-350.

Peck, M., and S. Jennings. (November 1989). "Student Perceptions of the Links Between Nursing and the Liberal Arts." *Journal of Nursing Education* 28(9): 406-414.

Read, J. (1980). "Alverno's Collegewide Approach to the Development of Valuing." In *Rethinking College Responsibilities for Values,* edited by M. McBee, 71-79. New Directions for Higher Education, no. 31. San Francisco, CA: Jossey-Bass.

Zaborowska, R. (April 1995). "Senior Nursing Students' Self-Reported College Experiences and Gains Toward Liberal Education Goals." *Journal of Nursing Education* 34(4): 155-161.

Preparing Nurses for Roles That Will Improve Community Health:
Two National Programs Enhance Relationships Between Providers and Educators

by Mary Kay Kohles, Maryalice Jordan-Marsh, and Margaret T. McNally

Setting the Stage

Service-learning, as it is linked to education, has been described by Kraft (1996) as having roots as diverse as Dewey's classic work in 1916 on one hand and the government Commission on National and Community Service on the other. These influences have been moderated by the constant American hunger for individualism but also reinforced by a "deep conviction that life has no meaning unless shared with others in the context of community" (Bellah et al. 1985). At present, service-learning is most pronounced within school systems (Kraft 1996), although there are many community-based examples (Shumer and Belbas 1996). As illustrated in this monograph series and in other reports (Headrick et al. 1995), the concept has been espoused at the college/university level, where it crosses both professional and basic science disciplines. More recently, the philosophy is emerging in health-care delivery systems that have undertaken restructuring. Service-learning is distinguished from other experiential learning, according to Furco (1996), by its balancing of benefits to the provider and to the recipient of the service while providing a simultaneous and equal focus on the service provided and the learning that results from it. Increasingly, incorporating the interests of those for whom the service is directed and empowering the recipients are proposed as core elements of service-learning (Maybach 1996). These elements form the basis of a new service-learning paradigm that provides context for designing health-care restructuring that is responsive to the consumer and recognizes the resources and strengths of that consumer and the community.

The views expressed in this essay are solely those of the authors. Official endorsement by the Robert Wood Johnson Foundation and the Pew Charitable Trusts is not intended and should not be inferred.

Furthermore, market reform is forcing reconsideration of the fundamental health-care mission, especially community health improvement, as consumers demand increasing value. Value in the new marketplace, as perceived by patients and payers, is defined by the equation:

$$Value = \frac{Clinical\ Quality \times Service\ Quality}{Cost}$$

While providers always have attempted to improve clinical quality and reduce costs, it is the new focus on services and the consumer perception of ease of access, convenience, match with expectations, and reasonable charges that characterizes many restructuring efforts today. This focus is more clearly delineated within a specific community served by providers and educators. Here "community" is understood as a geographic area such as a metropolitan area, rural region, a large neighborhood, or other areas defined by geographic boundaries (Healthcare Forum Leadership Center 1993) where people have commitments to one another (Farley 1986). Representative groups of providers, educators, and consumers from a community can come together for the common purpose of creating an environment that allows the members of the community to work toward a higher quality of life. Service-learning activities are one way these players can come together to focus on the common good.

Two national programs provide examples of implementing this new paradigm for health-care service from the standpoint of either restructuring the provider organization or redesigning the educational experience of the provider. Both programs stress the need for enhanced relationships among all involved parties, including educators and recipients of care or service. "Strengthening Hospital Nursing: A Program to Improve Patient Care" (SHNP) shows that attention to the needs of the patients and their families, rather than the needs of departments or disciplines, results in sustainable improvements in four key indicators of value: clinical outcomes, resource use, cost-benefit ratio, and satisfaction (patient, provider, payer, external review groups). "National Project Ladders in Nursing Careers" (L.I.N.C.) has focused on the relationship between providers and educators and has incorporated the changes taking place in health-care delivery into academic curricula through field experiences for nurses wishing to advance their careers.

Each program emphasizes establishing a balance between learning goals and service outcomes and provides opportunities for critical thinking and reflection among the involved parties.[1] The importance of structured opportunities for participants to critically think about their experiences and reflect on what they learned has been part of the implementation of the various projects that are represented in this chapter. It was through discussions and the critical reflection of the involved participants, including providers, educators, and consumers, that the group as a whole has been able to develop a stronger sense of social responsibility in and to a specific geographic community. This chapter will provide an overview of the efforts of the two national programs and illustrate examples of service-learning.

Overview of the Two National Programs

Both programs were conceived during the nursing shortage of the late 1980s, and both quickly recognized that changes in the health-care environment did not support efforts to recruit and retain nurses for the improvement of patient services. Hence, each program focused attention on what is valued by both providers and consumers, and value indicators were determined based on the equation presented earlier. Health-care delivery systems that are flexible, responsive, convenient, appropriate, and cost-effective are valued by both the provider and the consumer. Also, care givers must have knowledge and skills appropriate to the services required by the recipient in many different settings. Thus, practicing nurses require experience in community service settings that focus on health, including wellness and prevention, as well as in illness care. As the concept of health is currently being redefined, it includes the dynamic relationship between personal wellness and experienced components of living and working environments. Relevant components include, but are not limited to, quality education, adequate housing, availability of meaningful employment, access to job skills training and retraining, access to efficient public transportation, availability of recreational opportunities, healthy and clean physical environments, and access to health education and preventive services (Healthcare Forum Leadership Center 1993). Attention to health and illness achieves an optimal balance between learning goals for the nurse and care outcomes for the person receiving service. In accomplishing these goals, both programs have emphasized experiential learning, opportunities for participation of the group being served, and reflection on the experience.

Strengthening Hospital Nursing: A Program to Improve Patient Care

The Robert Wood Johnson Foundation and the Pew Charitable Trusts combined resources to fund a national grant to demonstrate that strengthening the use of existing professional resources, especially nursing, would improve cost-effective patient-care outcomes. They agreed that a fundamental change in the health-care delivery system might make it possible for nurses and other professionals to address problems that would create new opportunities for more efficient delivery of optimal patient-care services. They wanted to do more than provide short-term solutions to recruit and retain nurses; they wanted to change the fundamental way nurses, physicians, and others work together for the improvement of patient-care services in a variety of settings. Hence, they funded the five-year national program Strengthening Hospital Nursing: A Program to Improve Patient Care. Implicit in this call for a paradigm shift was the charge to recognize and engage the resources and strengths of the patients, families, and relevant communities. Twelve hospitals and six hospital consortia, representing more than 68 health-care organizations throughout the United States, participated in the five-year demonstration initiative.

Innovative models for efficiently and conveniently meeting the needs of patients and their families within and beyond hospital boundaries resulted from the efforts of 18 project teams. They demonstrated how collaborative care practices, case management, and integrated clinical delivery systems, concepts, and principles can support a shift of care from the hospital to a continuum of care across multiple service settings. Many of these innovations created new relationships between hospitals and educators that resulted in curricular changes and clinical experiences for students in nontraditional settings, such as long-term, home, clinic, and rural settings (Kohles et al. 1995). As wellness and prevention became priorities, these relationships also included community service organizations such as schools, parishes, and neighborhood health clinics. Student nurses receiving experience in these service settings were considered for hire as new graduates, promoting the reciprocal benefit resulting from the experience. SHNP officially ended in October 1995 (Strengthening Hospital Nursing 1996).

National Project Ladders in Nursing Careers

The Robert Wood Johnson Foundation also funded National Project Ladders in Nursing Careers. This project was designed to meet hospital nursing workforce needs by providing career ladder opportunities to entry- and mid-level health-care personnel already working within health-care settings. L.I.N.C. placed emphasis on minority and low-income individuals and established a strategy for meeting health-care agencies' projected needs for nurses. Three-year funding paved the way for L.I.N.C. participants to return to school by providing a comprehensive support system and financial resources for textbooks, enhancement courses including reading and mathematics, and other technical support to assist students in moving toward successful and satisfying careers. L.I.N.C. has provided the mechanism for students to attend school while maintaining employment. The student's tuition was supported by the institution employing the student or by financial resources from local community foundations or businesses. L.I.N.C.'s goals included preparing nurses for roles that will improve community health by stressing preparation of advanced-practice nurses for economically depressed regions and enrolling minority nurses for roles in leadership and clinical practice within areas that have a significant minority population. For example, states with Native American populations supported Native American students for clinical and leadership roles within their native health centers and other health-related service areas. L.I.N.C. was operationalized through eight state hospital associations or hospital foundations in Georgia, Iowa, Maryland, Minnesota, North Dakota, Rhode Island, South Carolina, and Texas. Funding ended in July 1997 (Project L.I.N.C. 1995).

The National Programs and Service-Learning

A synthesis of research over the past 20 years (Shumer and Belbas 1996) indicates that service-learning takes many forms, exemplary programs have regular dialogue among all parties, including organized reflection, the fun and pleasure of participation is an essential motive, and growth in self-esteem and social responsibility are frequent outcomes. SHNP and the L.I.N.C. program illustrate applications of these elements of service-learning targeted to health-care goals. In both cases, there was a recognition of the need to shift from care of individuals in specialized in-patient settings to an alternative paradigm addressing the "health of the public" (Seifer et al. 1996). Both programs designed clinical experiences for students and practicing nurses to learn in community-service settings, including parishes, schools, and health clinics, and emphasized the relationship between learning goals and service outcomes. While giving of their talents, these nurses and students increased their awareness about the needs and interests of individuals and groups in their specific geographic community. There was a mutual benefit for the nurse and the recipient of the service, as well as recognition that nursing curricula must change in order to prepare nurses for effective community service–related roles.

Both programs demonstrated that organ-based, disease-specific models of education and training are becoming less relevant as the basis for nursing knowledge and practice competencies than is the "reciprocal learning" that occurs at the point of a service setting. Traditional nursing education should be combined with practice experiences that address psychological and social approaches to health and illness, cultural and ethnic issues, and other demographic changes of the population affecting public health. As curricula and field experiences are collaboratively designed, providers and educators must be encouraged to redefine *health*, focusing on priority factors that undergird individual and community health and identifying the relationship between illness, wellness, and preventive measures (Healthcare Forum Leadership Center 1993; Kohles et al. 1995). They must be encouraged to join with civic groups, minority coalitions, and businesses in redefining health curricula and student experiences, ensuring that both the service recipient and the student are benefited by the mutual experience (Furco 1996). SHNP and L.I.N.C. supported the following core beliefs:

1. Nurse and student nurse learning can be enhanced through thoughtfully coordinated learning goals and service outcomes among the healthcare facilities, educational institutions, and service settings.

2. Different individual, social, cultural, and economic backgrounds may influence how nurses and students learn, including special tutoring and mentoring requirements.

3. Learning is an experiential process enhanced by critical thinking through reflection on application of knowledge and skills to real-life experiences.

4. Academic curriculum content and methods may need to change to meet the needs of nurses and students in their community, including providing distance learning and field experiences in nontraditional environments.

5. Descriptive research and assessment methods are essential components of demonstrating the impact for the nurse, student, organization, and service setting, and include keeping of journals, interviews of nurses, students, and recipients of service, and identification of quality and cost indicators.

6. Empowerment requires sustained dialogue with equal input from all players with a paradigm shift from provider-identified needs of the community to exploration of group-defined interests and agreement on mutual goals.

Highlights From SHNP and L.I.N.C. Projects

Highlights and examples of the interventions and outcomes of representative samples of both SHNP and L.I.N.C. projects follow, with emphasis on those interventions that relate to the concepts and principles of service-learning.

SHNP Projects

Some extant service-learning programs are coming under fire for being one-sided, with emphasis on benefits to the student without equal emphasis on the service recipient. In particular, Keith (1996) and others are calling for an adjustment where the input of the recipients is an essential element of program design. The hallmark for SHNP was the interactive planning and management structure implemented between educators and providers. This structure allowed both parties to identify a shared vision and implement interventions to achieve outcomes beneficial to their unique environments.

The strength of the structure was in its valuing of collaboration, its understanding of both parties' talents and knowledge, and its willingness to assess the impact on all affected by the interventions. This section will highlight four programs where dialogue between learners and recipients was a key feature. Three programs involved nurses and nursing students as the learners in service partnered with community agencies; in the fourth, the learners were medical center service providers who partnered with the patients.

• Health Bond, Mankato, Minnesota, a service and education partnership, developed a shared governance model to bring providers, educators, and consumers together for the purpose of designing opportunities to improve the health of people in south central Minnesota. Some of the projects resulting from their collaborative efforts were the Mankato Hilltop Neighbors Living at Home/Block Nurse Program, the Open Door Health Center, and the Faith-Health Ministry program. These projects gave priority to helping uninsured and underinsured individuals receive service in the most appropriate and cost-efficient environment, including the home, parish, and neighborhood. Each project allowed the nurse to learn about the most pressing needs of the person, design interventions for those needs, and implement methods to shift hospital-based care management to a continuum-of-care case management model.

• Abbott Northwestern Hospital, Minneapolis, Minnesota, designed the Home Town Nurse Program, in which a nurse from the hospital established a relationship with a small community, often her own, outside Minneapolis. This relationship was based on mutually defined goals of community nurse providers and Abbott Northwestern nurses along with recommendations from patients. Before becoming a Home Town Nurse, the nurse visited the community and spent time with other nurses from the local community hospital, home care, and other service centers where patients from that community receive health-related services, including psychological and social support, to develop an understanding of what the community can offer patients. If a patient from the community was admitted to Abbott Northwestern, the Home Town Nurse visited the patient and family and facilitated hospitality and other services to enhance patient comfort and identify specific outcomes to be achieved when he or she returned to the community, either to the local hospital, home, or another care setting. The nurse maintained a liaison relationship with the patient and family as long as there was a need perceived by the patient and served as the personal contact for questions and concerns from the patient, family, or community care providers once the patient was discharged from Abbott Northwestern. There was mutual benefit for the nurse giving care and the patient receiving care beyond clinical outcomes. The Home Town Nurse shared the knowledge she had learned about the services of the small community with other Abbott

Northwestern nurses. They in turn integrated care practices into their case management delivery model to support the unique aspects of this and other small communities.

• Tallahassee Memorial Regional Medical Center, Tallahassee, Florida, initiated a SHNP project that formed a partnership among community educators from all levels, including secondary, high school, and college/university, and health-care providers. This created a unique opportunity for students to have an apprenticeship at the hospital to observe nursing careers. Not only did potential and existing students develop an increased awareness of the value and satisfaction of a nursing career, but the partnership also resulted in significant changes in the nursing school curriculum that extended case management methodologies into community settings.

• Harbor-UCLA Medical Center, Torrance, California, is an example of service-learning from a very innovative perspective (Siler et al. 1995). In this project, introducing academic content specific to organizational change and promoting fun and enjoyment as legitimate work experiences were linked to strategies designed to build a sense of community among providers and patients as well as a sense of shared responsibility for organizational and clinical outcomes. The foundation of this effort was the goal of enhancing the medical center's internal community and all those who were embedded in commitments related to the center (patients, families, staff, students, vendors, neighbors, payers, etc.). The effort was begun by forming councils of executives, middle management, staff, and patients. Their task was to tackle projects and support the vision of a more effective organization that delivered patient-focused care. Projects undertaken by the councils included empowering nurses, children, and their families in pain management; improving triage in the emergency room; and testing a greeter program to humanize the 60-acre, 180-specialty, 500-bed hospital setting. These and other projects were accomplished using multiple strategies to optimize organizational learning (Jordan-Marsh et al. 1996; Wenger 1996). As a result of the shared educational and innovative experiences and reflection on the process, members saw opportunities for leadership, boundaries became more permeable, and a new willingness on the part of members to allow others to make claims on them emerged to create a *community of practice* (Drath and Palus 1994; Wenger 1996).

Across the 18 projects (only four of which are highlighted here), SHNP providers reported enhanced care giver and patient satisfaction, improved continuity of care between service environments, decreased length of hospital stay, decreased use of the emergency room, and significant cost savings. Student nurses indicated they felt they were being better prepared for future roles and felt they were a vital part of the care-giver team, contributing to care outcomes rather than merely being observer task managers. Educators are now making curriculum changes to include skills in creating and sustaining group dialogue, a more population-focused overall paradigm, and skills in initiating and sustaining organizational change. Providers, consumers, and educators agree that, while such changes are difficult, better value has been the outcome for all parties involved, particularly for patients and their families. In an era of scarce resources, partnerships like these draw more effectively on existing resources and, in some cases, generate a willingness to support new resources.

L.I.N.C. Projects

L.I.N.C. worked simultaneously at a macro and a micro level. At the macro level, it encouraged health-care facilities to think strategically about their long-term workforce needs and created a pipeline to meet those needs by bringing health-care institutions and schools together in the planning and implementation processes. Moreover, it allowed health-care institutions to tap into their existing employee base to meet future workforce needs — a benefit to employer and employee. L.I.N.C. also provided mechanisms for dialogue among employers, educators, and students, allowing for a more meaningful understanding of the relationship between health-service and workforce needs at a global level (Project L.I.N.C. 1995).

At the micro level, the importance of L.I.N.C. was demonstrated in the individual success of each and every student. The project provided an avenue for qualified individuals to obtain or further a nursing education. For advanced nursing students, it provided an opportunity to learn outside the traditional walls of the hospital, facilitating their ability to enhance quality of life for individuals receiving service and to improve community health (Project L.I.N.C. 1995). At this level, the needs of the service recipients were appraised and incorporated in the learning experiences of the students. Empowerment of and learning by recipients as well as students were core elements of the L.I.N.C. micro strategies. What follows highlights three of the eight L.I.N.C. projects where connections among hospitals, educational institutions, and community services or other service providers were key components.

• L.I.N.C. in Minnesota developed creative connections between a hospital and clinic in Faribault and Mankato State University in Mankato. A L.I.N.C. student's tuition was supported by the hospital where she was employed and the clinic where she would be employed as a family nurse practitioner. This reciprocal relationship allowed both the small community hospital and the clinic to have access to the services of a nurse practitioner, who would integrate practices from both settings as she coordinated the care of patients with other care providers. Part of her goal was to learn from the patient and family about their specific needs in order to design her practice. She observed the specific parenting and child development needs of the community through her interactions with mothers, school officials, parish contacts, and other community residents. She became familiar with the interests, priorities, and strengths of the community that were resources for meeting those needs.

• L.I.N.C. in Iowa initiated a forum bringing educators and providers together to identify workforce needs, concentrating on "homegrown" practitioners. Their partnership resulted in the development of continuing education strategies and field opportunities allowing experienced hospital nurses from large urban hospitals to learn new knowledge and skills in outpatient and community settings. They also identified strategies to provide rural community nurses opportunities for practice education and encouraged them to stay within the community supporting their educational efforts. Community service concepts and principles were integrated into nursing curricula, and field experiences were planned for nurses and students in service settings outside the hospital. Iowa has been successful in obtaining funds from a farming business to help support the scholarship needs of students seeking health career advancement. This support has heightened business awareness of health-care workforce needs and the contribution of "growing your own" workers. There is a belief by Iowa L.I.N.C. that through the reciprocal relationship among the involved parties, these workers will be stable and consistent in promoting the community's culture and values. Educators, providers, and businesses have identified health workforce requirements based on mutual assessment and have planned strategies to support those needs, particularly on the shift of services from hospitals to ambulatory and community service settings.

• L.I.N.C. in North Dakota brought together representatives from the University of North Dakota medical and nursing schools and Blue Cross/Blue Shield of North Dakota and included providers in rural and urban settings to explore the feasibility of using telemedicine and videoconferencing to create new opportunities for nursing students to advance their careers through long-distance learning mechanisms. This reciprocal relationship heightened awareness of existing local community needs and resulted in curricular redesign to tailor learning to meet those needs.

A hallmark of L.I.N.C. is the core belief that an education counselor serves as an advocate for her student, negotiating and facilitating issues that might interfere with the student's career advancement goals. For example, the student's work schedule may interfere with the student's attending class. The counselor will negotiate a more acceptable schedule, mutually beneficial to the student and employer. In other cases, the academic curriculum has been adjusted to accommodate students from different ethnic and cultural backgrounds, particularly stressing language skills and understanding of terminology. Many L.I.N.C. students have indicated they would not have been able to pursue an advanced nursing career without L.I.N.C. support, and they appreciated the opportunity to improve not only their own quality of life and that of their families but also the quality of life of the communities they serve. Educators likewise have indicated they are now more sensitive to the needs and interests of students presenting ethnic and cultural differences and have made curricular changes based on those insights. Providers and educators agree that forming partnerships has facilitated the drafting of implementable strategies to meet both community and workforce needs.

Challenges for the Future

The intent of this chapter has been to illustrate nurse-initiated projects as examples of successful service-learning. The projects have in common a respect for diversity, an emphasis on input and dialogue among the partners, the practice of reflection on both process and outcome, an interdisciplinary approach, and an expectation that all participants are learners. Among the lessons learned were the value of fully appreciating the resources and strengths of both the formal health-care experts and the community members, the fact that each participant is both learner and teacher, and the fact that innovations cannot be totally dependent on grant funding if they are to influence continued improvements for creating an environment that brings health-care providers and educators together for the purpose of enhancing quality of life for a given community. Through their discussions, which include critical reflection on past and present efforts, they will influence our redefinition of health, placing greater emphasis on the value of prevention.

The details of these implementations and specific lessons learned are beyond the scope of this chapter; interested readers are referred to the reference section. However, based on the combined experiences of the programs in these two national initiatives, it seems clear that the service-learning literature has much to offer consumers, organizations, educators, and health-care delivery systems in planning for the future. The core competencies identified in 1991 by the Pew Health Professions Commission report (Shugars et al. 1991) — practicing prevention, promoting healthy life-styles, and involving patients and their families in health-care decision making — continue to be relevant. Based on the experiences discussed above, even greater emphasis needs to be given to the recommendations of the 1995 Pew Health Professions Commission report for developing competencies in using sophisticated information and communications technology, facilitating political reforms, becoming consumer-focused, and being able to balance needs and resources.

The value equation presented at the beginning of this essay will be an increasingly important component not only in determining the worth of health-care services in the marketplace but also in evaluating the impact of service-learning models. In an ideal service-learning effort, providers, educators, and consumers together seek out opportunities to understand what they should be doing to improve the health status of the community. They influence the redefinition of health, placing an emphasis on the value of prevention, maintenance, and wellness services, particularly those services that promote public health and the quality of life for all individuals.

Service-learning-oriented relationships among providers, educators, and consumers have tremendous potential. However, research and evaluation methodologies need to be developed to show the impact of service-learning for preceptors, students, educators, and the partner-recipients of the service. This work will be expedited by a common definition of service-learning and a commitment from participants to contribute to the national database. Finally, over time, it is in the interest of all parties to blur the boundaries between what is traditionally referred to as the community where service is delivered and the settings that send forth the learners/providers. The ultimate goal is a community of practice where leadership is shared and members make common sense (Drath and Palus 1994).

Note

1. The following references provide additional information about the 18 grantees participating in SHNP: Hanson and Sayers 1995; Kohles, Baker, and Donaho 1995; and Schmeling 1995. Additional information about SHNP can be obtained from Barbara A. Donaho, program director, at 813/522-6433 or Mary K. Kohles, deputy director, at 404/605-2453. Additional information about Project L.I.N.C. can be obtained from Margaret T. McNally at 212/246-7100.

References

Bellah, R., R. Madsen, W. Sullivan, A. Swidler, and S. Tipton. (1985). *Habits of the Heart*. Berkeley, CA: University of California Press.

Drath, W.H., and C.J. Palus. (1994). *Making Common Sense: Leadership as Meaning-Making in a Community of Practice*. Greensboro, NC: Center for Creative Leadership.

Farley, M. (1986). *Personal Commitments*. San Francisco, CA: Harper & Row.

Furco, A. (January 1996). "Service-Learning: A Balanced Approach to Experiential Education." In *Expanding Boundaries: Serving and Learning,* 2-6. Washington, DC: Corporation for National Service.

Hanson, R.B., and B. Sayers. (1995). *Work and Role Redesign: Tools and Techniques for the Health Care Setting.* Chicago, IL: American Hospital Publishing.

Headrick, L., L. Norman, S. Gelmon, and M. Knapp. (August 29, 1995). *Interdisciplinary Professional Education in the Continuous Improvement of Health Care: The State of the Art.* Final report. Health Services Resources Administration, Bureau of the Health Professions.

Healthcare Forum Leadership Center's Healthier Communities Partnership. (1993). *Healthier Communities Action Kit: A Guide for Leaders Embracing Change.* Module 1. San Francisco, CA: Healthcare Forum.

Jordan-Marsh, M., P. Nazarey, P. Siler, S.R. Goldsmith, and E. Sanchez. (1996). "Structural Innovations and Transitions for the Nurse Executive in the Change Agent Role." In *The Executive Nurse: Leadership for New Health Care Transitions,* edited by S. Beyers, 84-94. Albany, NY: Delmar.

Keith, N.Z. (January 1996). "Can Urban School Reform and Community Development Be Joined? The Potential of Community Schools." *Education and Urban Society* 28(1): 237-268.

Kohles, M.K., W.G. Baker, and B.A. Donaho. (1995). *Transformational Leadership: Renewing Fundamental Values and Achieving New Relationships in Health Care.* Chicago, IL: American Hospital Publishing.

Kraft, R.J. (February 1996). "Service-Learning: An Introduction to Its Theory, Practice, and Effects." *Education and Urban Society* 28(2): 131-159.

Maybach, C.W. (February 1996). "Investigating Urban Community Needs: Service-Learning From a Social Justice Perspective." *Education and Urban Society* 28(2): 224-236.

Pew Health Professions Commission. (1995). *Critical Challenges: Revitalizing the Health Professions for the Twenty-first Century.* San Francisco, CA: UCSF Center for the Health Professions.

Project L.I.N.C. (1995). *Building Bridges: A Progress Report* [of the Ladders in Nursing Careers Program, the Robert Wood Johnson Foundation]. New York, NY: National Program Office, Greater New York Hospital Foundation.

Schmeling, W. (1995). *Facing Change in Health Care: Learning Faster in Tough Times.* Chicago, IL: American Hospital Publishing.

Seifer, S.D., S. Mutha, and K. Connors. (January 1996). "Service-Learning in Health Professions Education: Barriers, Facilitators, and Strategies for Success." In *Expanding Boundaries: Serving and Learning,* 36-41. Washington, DC: Corporation for National Service.

Shugars, D.A., E.H. O'Neil, and J.D. Bader, eds. (1991). *Survey of Practitioners' Perceptions of Their Education.* Durham, NC: Pew Health Professions Commission.

Shumer, R., and B. Belbas. (February 1996). "What We Know About Service-Learning." *Education and Urban Society* 28(2): 131-159.

Siler, P.V., M. Jordan-Marsh, P. Nazarey, S.R. Goldsmith, and E. Sanchez. (1995). "The Community Design Model: A Framework for Restructuring." In *Series on Nursing Administration*. Vol. 7, *Health-Care Work Redesign*. Edited by K. Kelly, 131-149. Thousand Oaks, CA: Sage.

Strengthening Hospital Nursing: A Program to Improve Patient Care. (1996). *Celebrating the Journey: A Final Report.* St. Petersburg, FL: National Program Office, All Children's Research Institute.

Wenger, E. (1996). "Communities of Practice: The Social Fabric of a Learning Organization." *Healthcare Forum* 39(4): 20-26.

Service Education Partnerships Create Community Service–Learning Opportunities in a Rural Region

by Sharon P. Aadalen, Mary Kay Hohenstein, Mary I. Huntley, and Annette J. McBeth

Extreme pendulum swings characterize the history of American nursing education and practice in this century. The nursing profession has experienced the limitations of apprenticeship in hospital training schools (Ashley 1976) and the relative isolation of ivory tower education in colleges and universities (Rush 1992). During the last two decades of the 20th century, a variety of initiatives have breathed life into efforts to integrate nursing education and nursing practice for advancing the health of individuals, families, populations, and communities, and knowledge building in the profession. Examples of these initiatives include the National Commission on Nursing Implementation Project (NCNIP 1990), Strengthening Hospital Nursing: A Program to Improve Patient Care (SHNP 1992-1995), the Teagle Foundation's LPN-to-BSN Initiative (1996), and the Ladders in Nursing Careers (L.I.N.C.) program (Greater New York 1996). These efforts have stressed the importance of autonomous nursing practice for leadership in community health and preparing nurses for effective interdisciplinary practice and consumer-responsive health care. The NCNIP, SHNP, LPN-BSN, and L.I.N.C. program emphases reflect Boyer's call (1990) for an integration of four categories of scholarship (research, synthesis, practice, and teaching). These initiatives have advanced strategies that reflect service-learning practices prevalent in K-12 education and liberal studies in higher education.[1] Such strategies transcend prior education- or practice-based initiatives, and create a new model of critical, reflective inquiry and praxis in which learning, practice, and community service are fully synthesized.

The views expressed in this essay are solely those of the authors. Official endorsement by the Robert Wood Johnson Foundation and the Pew Charitable Trusts, Mankato State University, South Central Technical College, and Immanual–St. Joseph's Hospital, Mayo Health System, is not intended and should not be inferred.

Contributors include Delight White, RN, BSN, program supervisor, Hilltop Neighbors LAH/BNP, Immanuel–St. Joseph's Hospital, Mayo Health System; Laura Rydholm, RN, MS, parish nurse facilitator, Immanuel–St. Joseph's Hospital, Mayo Health System; Susan Frost, RN, BSN, nurse case manager, Maternal Child Home Care, Immanuel–St. Joseph's Hospital, Mayo Health System, and nurse manager, ODHC; and Debra Thompson, RN, C, BSN, instructor, MSU School of Nursing, and nurse manager, ODHC.

Health Bond Consortium: The Setting

Health Bond is a voluntary, noncontractual rural service-education partnership of three member hospitals (Arlington Municipal Hospital, Waseca Area Memorial Hospital, and Immanuel–St. Joseph's Hospital) and two partner higher education institutions (Mankato State University and South Central Technical College) located in a nine-county south central Minnesota region. The Health Bond Consortium was one of 18 projects in the SHNP initiative, funded by the Robert Wood Johnson Foundation and the Pew Charitable Trusts. This service-education consortium envisioned providing quality, cost-effective patient- and family-centered care, redesigning and integrating health-care services, and becoming the providers and employers of choice for people in the region.

Key elements that created the foundation for Health Bond included interdisciplinary interactive visioning and planning, consumer-centered services, quality cost-effective health care, and systems thinking. Consortium members designed a shared governance structure to operationalize the service-education partnership. Consultation and education emphasizing skill building focused on concepts of communication, relationship management, leadership development, empowerment, primary-care delivery, and collaborative decision making.

In the years prior to the formation of the Health Bond Consortium, the culture and climate within and among service and education organizations and the community were not hospitable to innovation. These systems appeared closed to the external environment, and they were. Developing healthy organizational and interorganizational cultures that support innovative design and implementation has been a major focus of the consortium.

Health Bond's vision, structure, and process guided the accomplishment of five objectives that have resulted in the development of a variety of community-based innovations. These objectives were to (1) promote cultural change among members of the health-care team to facilitate continuous quality improvement, (2) integrate a regional network of service and education providers, (3) develop indicators to measure improvement in the quality and cost-effectiveness of care and service throughout the redesign process, (4) improve coordination of services to promote a continuum of patient- and family-centered health care, and (5) provide leadership through an interactive planning process for developing a regional health-care system responsive to rural consumers.

In the course of opening a door to providing creative leadership for quality, cost-effective health-care and education services in a rural region, a profound kind of service-learning has evolved: *a collaboration model* developed by service and education representatives working together to create trustworthy partnerships around shared goals. In 1988, consortium planners did not start with a clear conceptualization of or intent to apply deductively a model of service-learning. Rather, using an inductive, ecological, experiential, action research–oriented approach, Health Bond participants sought to expand their own thinking and gain new understanding of their work by participating in learning teams. In the process, they began opening the door for health-care consumers, providers, and staff to manage their own health as individuals and groups. Students, as faculty colleagues, began assuming more responsibility for their individual and collective learning.

$$1 + 1 = > 2$$

The whole is greater than the sum of its parts.

New programs, such as the Hilltop Neighbors Living at Home/Block Nurse Program, a senior citizen health center, the Faith-Health Ministry, the Open Door Health Center, and the Regional Continuing Healthcare Education Council (ReCHEC), flowed out of the Health Bond Consortium objectives related to integrating a regional network of service and education providers for leadership in family- and consumer-oriented health care.

New models of nurse-managed interdisciplinary care and education in the community combined skilled nursing (staff, faculty, and students) and lay volunteers along with other providers and clients to allow underserved populations access to empowering health care and education. One outcome has been the creation of new service-learning opportunities.

Service-Learning: Innovations and Outcomes

Roles of clients (health-care consumers and students) and providers (clinicians, managers, and faculty) are changing, just as the major paradigms in health care and the greater environment are changing. Good people working together are creating learning organizations in which people are helping one another move forward.

When clients and staff experience health services reflecting the concepts of freedom, trust, and caring, there is a fertile environment for service-learning (Aadalen et al. 1996; Aadalen et al. 1997; McBeth and Weydt 1996). Everyone thrives when service-learning opportunities create what Parker Palmer (1995) describes as a "capacity for connectedness." Such opportunities open a space for compassion and enable faculty, students, clients, and nursing and other professional staff to become "smarter faster."

Outcomes of Health Bond Consortium interdisciplinary service/education and volunteer staff partnership development activities demonstrate service-learning opportunities created through the stages of planning, implementing, strengthening, maintaining, and replicating community-based innovations in health care. These outcomes would not have occurred without the penetrating reflection and honest description of the current realities of problematic health care and relationships between education and service providers by a committed interdisciplinary group of providers.

Hilltop Neighbors Living at Home/Block Nurse Program

Health Bond sponsored an information session for south central Minnesota in the fall of 1991 in which community leaders heard about start-up funding available through the state legislature for seven rural Minnesota Living at Home/Block Nurse Programs (LAH/BNPs). Several participants in this session formed a planning group with other community members to develop a grant proposal. This proposal was one of the seven funded. Community-based, these programs draw upon the professional and volunteer services of local residents to provide information, social and support services, skilled nursing, and other services to their neighbors aged 65 and older to enable them to remain safely in their own homes. Each LAH/BNP defines its own geographic neighborhood. The Mankato Hilltop neighborhood represents the highest concentration (24%) of Mankato residents 65 years and older, compared with the city of Mankato, with 10.9 percent of individuals 65 years and older.

Each LAH/BNP depends on grass-roots community interest in and the active commitment of service groups, churches, businesses, and schools. Mankato Hilltop Neighbors LAH/BNP includes four churches, three elementary schools, a junior and senior high school, a two-year private college and nearby university, a major regional health center and a large multispecialty physician practice, two large shopping centers, two major supermarkets, many banks and restaurants, and other businesses. The neighborhood also includes three senior housing facilities, one public, one occupant-owned, and one private. Many volunteers have been recruited through the churches, schools, service groups such as the Moose, and the hospital and other health-care providers.

The financial base of support for the Hilltop Neighbors Living at Home/Block Nurse Program is diverse, including federal and state grant funds, local community and business contributions, and the in-kind and financial support of the regional health center that is in the neighborhood. The LAH/BNP pays for services not covered by Medicare or Medicaid through community fundraising. The program bills clients according to their ability to pay and provides services regardless of client ability to pay or eligibility for reimbursement. The program provides free service if indicated.

The program in Mankato has two neighborhood Block Nurses who provide skilled nursing, case management, and supervision of home health aides/homemakers. These two nurses work with nursing students from the school of nursing at the local university, who may be community health nursing students doing clinicals, nursing leadership or long-term care internship students, graduate students exploring nurse-managed community nursing programs, or students in health sciences or community health doing a variety of clinical studies. These students have the opportunity to acquire, through these planned curricular experiences, a vision of how they will fulfill their own mission as a nurse where they live as well as where they work. Through these experiences, students reflect on the importance to senior citizens of being able to remain in their homes, gaining a whole new appreciation of the meaning of "activities of daily living" for people 65 years and older dealing with the health challenges of chronic disease. They come to understand the kind of skilled nursing and volunteer services necessary to enable these people to manage their health challenges in their home community, and they discover some of the stark economic realities many elderly people face. As students process their experiences, they discover the power of people in community working together to mobilize their own strength and their resources, and to solve their own problems.

Since Mankato Hilltop Neighbors LAH/BNP began providing services in March 1993, program participants have served 270 older neighbors, and 138 persons have received home-care nursing services. These statistics are conservative and represent unduplicated services. During the past two years, the total estimated health cost savings due to the Mankato Hilltop LAH/BNP was $718,647. This calculation is based on actual program costs and estimated nursing home costs.

The ultimate goals of LAH/BNPs are to design an appropriate combined service coordination and delivery model for meeting the long-term needs of the elderly that is home- and community-based/focused, and to create a new and more inclusive system for paying for long-term care. This program is an excellent example of nursing's natural leadership emerging in interdisciplinary projects and initiatives based on nursing education and experience related to care coordination (LAH/BNP newsletters 1993-1996).

Senior Citizen Health Clinic

Within the geographic neighborhood of the Hilltop Neighbors Living at Home/Block Nurse Program is a Housing and Urban Development (HUD)–supported senior citizen residence. Collaboration among the Hilltop Neighbors LAH/BNP, the housing authority, and two faculty members from Mankato State University's School of Nursing (a member of the community health faculty and a faculty member expert in gerontological nursing) resulted in the creation of a community-based nursing clinic for seniors. The clinic, staffed by MSU nursing students, their instructors, and LAH/BNP volunteers, is housed at a high-rise complex in the Mankato Hilltop area. The faculty members combined their groups of junior gerontology and senior community health students in order to provide blood pressure screening, medication review, hospital discharge follow-up, and basic nursing assessments for residents.

The more experienced community health nursing students mentored the gerontology nursing students. When junior-year students in the gerontology course had the opportunity to return to the clinic the following year in their community health practicum, they experienced a change in the seniors who came to the clinic. As they reflected on their experience and the clients they were working with, they realized the change was in themselves and how they saw people 65 and older. The student perceptions of client capability expanded considerably between the students' third and fourth years in the baccalaureate program. Pairs of students made "home visits" to residents who could not come to the clinic. Equipment donated by the regional health center and private cash donations from the community made it possible for the students to offer two special procedures, foot care and ear washing, at no charge to clinic users.

The clinic eventually was made available to other senior citizens from the Hilltop area. Clinic hours were 9-11:30 am. On clinic days, the nursing students stayed into the afternoon in order to organize a "social hour." During this hour, the students provided health education and created opportunities for those attending to reminisce about their lives and experiences. Donations from a grocery store allowed the students to provide healthy snacks and beverages for the group.

Residents who have participated in the clinic are very enthusiastic and experience significant support from the clinic program. Students are most impressed with the abilities of the senior citizens. Those students who have had the opportunity for this service-learning experience in their junior gerontology course and again in their senior community health nursing course have observed growth and development in the relationships and caring demonstrated by the residents among themselves. Reflecting on these changes in previously isolated seniors, students have had mirrored back to them the power of autonomous nursing care. Students appreciate the opportunity to return to the clinic during their senior clinical rotations. They value the influence this experience has had on defining the scope of professional nursing practice for themselves. Returning as senior nursing students, they have been very impressed with the residents' responses, the growth of the clinic program, and the increasing numbers of seniors participating.

Approximately 178 Hilltop seniors have been served at the clinic since September 1994. The community-based senior citizen health clinic is open one day per week in this one site during student clinical rotations. Other nursing faculty members have expressed interest in expanding this service-learning opportunity to other junior and senior nursing students through developing other clinic sites. Faculty are recognizing the potential of the model for replication in many other areas of health needs in the community.

Faith-Health Ministry: Parish Nursing

In 1992, an interdisciplinary Faith-Health Ministries Innovation project team comprising clergy, hospital nursing personnel, and school of nursing faculty successfully competed for Health Bond Consortium small-grant funding to send a team of people to an educational program in Chicago. A sequel to this "new beginning" was the establishment and funding of a part-time position of parish nursing facilitator by the regional health center. Parish nurses are ministers of health to congregations. The parish nursing facilitator sees herself as a parish nurse to 90 nurses who serve 50 church-es in a nine-county south central Minnesota region.

Parish nurses contribute their time and efforts to helping parishioners resolve concerns that threaten their well-being. Some parish nurses work in remote areas in small parish settings. Others are working in larger church settings as part of a six- to eight-member parish nurse team. Many parish nurses are employed in other settings in service and education. Other parish nurses are students in the RN-to-BSN program or graduate advanced-prac-tice nursing program at the school of nursing. They describe their voluntary service as a parish nurse as very meaningful and a stimulus to their growth as a person and as a nurse. The service-learning opportunity provided by parish nursing exemplifies the holism of the mind, body, and spirit, inte-grated and indivisible. Processing this experience in groups facilitated by the parish nursing coordinator for the region and by faculty encourages nurses working in parishes to reflect on and claim their newly discovered freedom to nurse. Being a parish nurse impacts the professional and personal lives of the nurses as well as those of their clients in remarkable ways.

Stories related to their experiences reflect both the need for their pres-ence and the cost-effectiveness of their interventions. As part of a grant funded through the regional development commission's Area Agency on Aging Funds, parish nurses describe interventions that have reduced their clients' risk of suffering an acute illness progression and are documenting client outcomes using DIARY notes (Data, Interpretation, Action, Response, and Yield documentation of interactions with a client). The parish nurse facilitator is working with nursing schools to computerize this documenta-tion using North American Nursing Diagnosis Association (NANDA 1996), the Iowa Nursing Interventions Classification (McCloskey and Bulecheck 1996), and the Iowa Nursing Outcomes Classification (Johnson and Maas 1997) systems.

Through this Faith-Health Ministry parish nurse program, participants not only are providing a very important service related to the health of rural parishioners (many of whom are elderly) but also are participating in the development of a significant documentation system for describing the role of parish nurses and demonstrating interventions and their effectiveness through carefully defined outcomes.

During the initial five-month period of parish nurse facilitation, an estimated $400,000 in health-care costs was avoided due to the timely and effective intervention of parish nurses. Rydholm (1997) reports that half of this estimated cost savings was due to interventions that supported and sustained care givers to facilitate ongoing home care. The other half of the estimated cost savings related to interventions that helped parishioners be more attentive to signs and symptoms of health problems that require medical attention. In a 1995 communication to Congressman David Minge from southwestern and south central Minnesota, Fernando Torres-Gil, the assistant secretary on aging, noted, "This project [south central Minnesota parish nursing facilitation] illustrates the savings and benefits that can be achieved through home- and community-based care."

Open Door Health Center

March 1996 marked the second anniversary of health services offered by the Open Door Health Center (ODHC), a nurse-managed service in Mankato, Minnesota. This center is the outcome of the vision and planning of a dedicated community-based interdisciplinary group of individuals, organizations, and agencies:

- Council for Health Action and Promotion
- county public health department
- regional development commission
- university school of nursing
- district representative of professional nursing organization
- Planned Parenthood clinic
- regional health center
- county medical society
- wellness center
- primary-care physician (leader in holistic health)
- chiropractor
- advanced-practice nurse
- dentist
- dental hygiene faculty
- university dental hygiene program.

The Open Door is a prevention- and wellness-oriented health center designed to meet the health needs of underserved people, especially women and children. The goal is to move to a new paradigm and model of care, a center for family health. As a nurse-managed center, the Open Door access-es clients to community-based interdisciplinary care and builds needed net-works that enhance resources on behalf of clients.

The health services and education provided by the Open Door Health Center encourage individuals and families to be involved in and responsible for their own health. The Open Door complements existing health services; it is not in competition with them. When client or family needs are beyond the scope of the center, the volunteer professional staff at Open Door serve referral, brokering, and triage functions to access clients to appropriate care and services.

The Open Door Health Center philosophy is grounded in the belief that all people should be able to access health-related services that are afford-able, appropriate, safe, and effective. Nurse-managed care is a holistic model of care. All services that can be provided by nurses are provided by nurses. Nursing care includes health assessments, education and information, time to answer any questions a person may have about his/her health, and sup-port so patients can be as healthy as possible. Nurses — including staff nurs-es, faculty, nurse clinicians, nurse practitioners, and students — relish the experience of practicing what they describe as *real* nursing at the center yet acknowledge the difficulty they have letting go of the medical model. At the center, their consciousness is raised about the underutilization of their pro-fessional knowledge, competence, and skill in some care-giving settings. Questions about the curriculum in nursing education programs are pro-voked. When patients tell nurses they like coming to the center because they are accepted fully, nurses are challenged to ponder the factors that make patients feel unaccepted, and therefore unsafe, in other settings.

If a person needs to see a nurse practitioner or other advanced-practice nurse, physician, nutritionist, dentist, dental hygienist, or provider of com-plementary modalities or therapies, the nurse arranges for that service. When nurses serve as brokers for clients to get into needed medical services, they begin to see discrimination that profoundly impacts access to health and medical care services for uninsured and underinsured citizens in the community. The fee at the Open Door Health Center is $5.00 per visit. No one is denied services if he/she is unable to pay. Services provided at the Open Door Health Center include:

- complete health history and physical examination
- limited care of common illnesses
- throat culture test to detect streptococcal infections
- dental screening, hygiene, and referral for children and youth up to age 18
- child and teen checkups
- developmental screening for children under 6 years of age

- measurement of height, weight, blood pressure, pulse, respirations
- screening of vision and hearing
- health education and counseling regarding individual concerns, particularly in relation to nutrition, exercise, development, family relations, or stress management
- immunizations
- health education
- referral to a primary-care provider or other resource for problems identified that are beyond the scope of the center.

Services that are not provided include comprehensive lab work, EKGs, X rays, or special studies.

Client consent and confidentiality are assured. If Open Door is referring a client to other services, the client signs a consent form so the needed information can be sent. The Open Door Health Center is open Tuesday and Thursday 3-6:00 pm and Wednesday 5-8:00 pm. The regional health center, county public health department, and university school of nursing have contributed professional nursing time and administrative support to the management function and nurse practitioner service at the center. All other personnel at the center are volunteers.

A profile of services provided June 1, 1994, to June 1, 1996, through the Open Door Health Center has been developed. The total number of clients seen was 1,752. This total does not include the 717 clients seen by public health nurses through the Public Health Teen/Child Check-up Clinic held at Open Door. The major reasons patients came to the Open Door Health Center were for prevention (immunizations and screening, health assessments and physical examinations, and wellness care) (63%) and treatment for acute conditions (32%), especially for diagnosis and treatment of upper respiratory infections. Most interventions (1,186, or 67%) were by nurses. Four hundred sixty-four clients (26%) required interventions by providers representing different disciplines, including nurse practitioners, physicians, dentists and hygienists, or mental health clinicians. Most patients were walk-ins (812, or 46%), while 516 (30%) made appointments in advance. Another 282 clients (16%) called ahead the same day for service. Clients used Open Door for the following reasons:
- uninsured — 698 (40%)
- underinsured — 466 (27%)
- convenience — 292 (17%)
- no physician — 96 (6%)
- unable to get care elsewhere — 73 (4%).

Most patients learned about the Open Door Health Center through:
- relative/friend — 407
- school nurse — 201

- doctor/nurse — 121
- newspaper — 118
- human services department — 93
- brochure — 58.

Over the first two years, two of the nine counties in the region were the source of the most clients. However, the Open Door Health Center has had clients from each of the nine counties (86% of clients come from this region) as well as clients from Minnesota locales outside the region, two other states, and at least five foreign countries (high school foreign exchange students or college- and graduate-level international students).

Service-learning opportunities have been available to state university students since the initial planning phase for the initiative. For example, a senior nursing student helped develop, administer, and analyze a needs assessment survey as part of her synthesis or capstone course learning experience in the nursing curriculum. This survey was distributed to 290 potential clients at sites such as food shelves, WIC clinics, the Salvation Army, and county health and financial services offices. There were 176 respondents. Sixty-three (63) percent said they, or their children, had not received medical services when they thought they had needed them in the past year. Fourteen (14) percent said they had been denied medical care in the past year. Sixty-two (62) percent of respondents reported three areas in which they needed services in the past year but for which they received no care: influenza and respiratory problems; bone, joint, and arthritis problems; and dental care. Of respondents to the survey, 14 percent had been denied medical services because of inability to pay, 27 percent always took their children with them to an appointment, 54 percent could not always afford to get their prescriptions filled, and 24 percent missed appointments due to transportation problems. Major barriers to care were cost/inability to pay, child care, and transportation issues.

Infants from 1 week through teens 18 years of age were 52 percent (914) of all clients served at the Open Door Health Center. Future plans include involving faculty and undergraduate and graduate students along with consumers to develop plans to meet the needs of this underserved population (infants, children, and teenagers). Simultaneously, School of Nursing faculty with pediatric and adolescent expertise are working with others in the community to develop integrated plans including curricular components to build assets in the youth of the community and region.

Health science students from Mankato State University have contracted to do internships at the Open Door Health Center. A student with a major in nursing who has a minor in community health served an internship at the Open Door Health Center. This student worked closely with a community dentist to help implement the dental screening, assessment, and cleaning program for children and youth up to the age of 18 years. Specific services include examinations, X rays, fluoride treatments, sealants, dental cleaning, and referrals. When the needs assessment survey was done, potential clients rated dental services as a very high need (six points on a seven-point scale) equaled only by identified needs related to upper respiratory infections. The dental program (5 to 8:30 pm on Tuesdays) began in September 1995 and is a very busy service. Dental hygiene students working with their supervisors and volunteer dentists from the community provide this service as a structured part of their curriculum. Eligible children are those who have no medical assistance, no dental insurance, and no Minnesota Care coverage. The fee is $5.00 per child or a donation. Nobody is turned away due to the inability to pay.

Beginning in 1995-96, nurse practitioners from the state university school of nursing faculty have worked at the Open Door Health Center as part of their faculty assignment. Graduate students from the state university's master's program have begun having clinical experiences at the Open Door Health Center, where faculty nurse practitioners serve as mentors/preceptors in their practitioner role at the center. The first rural family nurse practitioner advanced-practice students obtained their master of science in nursing degrees in June 1996. Several of these nurse practitioners are eager to volunteer at Open Door.

Regional Continuing Healthcare Education Council

Beginning in 1992, the Regional Continuing Healthcare Education Council (ReCHEC) evolved from the Education and Information Standing Committee of the Health Bond Consortium shared governance structure. Representatives from the state university, regional health center, and technical college began to meet to develop a long-range plan to meet the education needs of nurses through an integrated network of service and education. Health Bond service and education partners, in providing continuing professional education, invited colleagues from the region representing long-term care, rural primary-care hospitals from the state department of health, and the state institution for the mentally ill and retarded to join them in developing a vision of collaborative continuing professional education for nurses essential to achieving excellence in health care.

The enlarged advisory committee quickly expanded the scope of the group's focus to the education of health-care personnel. The ReCHEC group defined a service-learning opportunity and challenge for its members: a need for a current assessment of the learning needs of nurses and allied health professionals in the nine-county region. These two surveys were conducted during succeeding summers and accomplished through commitments of member time, institutional in-kind support, and a small grant from

Health Bond.

Participation in this group has changed the thinking of the service and education provider members. They have successfully written grants together to further their mission of providing collaborative learning opportunities to enhance high-quality care. One service provider said in 1994,

> One of our original goals was to plan and implement a physical center for nursing and nursing education in this region. In the 18 months [since ReCHEC members began meeting], many other factors, such as the Healthcare Reform Plan, have impacted our discussions. But a center exists in our mental and emotional images that encourages us to work together to provide educational opportunities to all health-care workers in our region. Together we will offer that education in the most efficient and cost-effective manner with a degree of quality that few of us could accomplish working alone.

Members of ReCHEC have come to appreciate that when they provide customized educational offerings, they as educators from service and education settings are learning about meeting community need, about the significance of their connections and linkages in the community, and about their accountability to the community. Each person takes this heightened awareness back to his or her respective worksite and home community, and becomes an influencer of others in the power of service-learning opportunities and experiences.

In the winter of 1996, a service and education team from the ReCHEC group went to a continuing professional education meeting on distance learning in another part of the country. They were very surprised to find themselves somewhat of an anomaly at the meeting. "You work together as service and education partners on a regular basis?!" For them, the most natural thing in the world is to be in a service-education partnership working on a common goal for the good of health professionals in their home region. However, this new identity, an identity of "us, ReCHEC service and education partners," was forged only because individuals, representing different organizations, risked stepping forward and meeting face-to-face to dream about a better future of continuing professional education in a nine-county rural region. The process was not easy; old competitiveness dies hard. The ReCHEC members were willing to reflect on where they had been, where they were, and where they were going at each meeting. This reflection was reinforcing; the strengths of their partnerships outweighed the barriers to their partnering. And each participant was changing in the process. The ReCHEC members returned home from the meeting with a heightened consciousness of the significance of their partnership and its enormous value to them. They are realizing their shared vision: that by 1997 ReCHEC would be the major role model for collaborative education essential for achieving excellence in health care.

The second "aha" for them was the change in their thinking from the idea of creating some kind of a physical center for nursing to creating a "virtual" continuing professional education community in the region. The group plans to use some of the grant money it has obtained to purchase portable computers and educational software that will be loaned to rural health-care provider systems on a rotating basis, thus accessing their colleagues who practice in relatively isolated settings with very limited staff to current significant educational resources in their own communities.

Service-Learning: Practical Considerations

Structural and process innovations that Health Bond partners found invaluable and essential precursors to nurturing the creation of new programs and models of health care in the community are described below. As these structures and processes were developed, opportunities were created for students from many disciplines within partner educational institutions to become involved through the curriculum in service-learning activities.

Interactive Planning Process

The interactive planning process advanced by Ackoff (1989) is a process for creating and managing change in complex social systems and is based on two essential concepts: systems thinking and design. Systems thinking provides a way of defining problems in organizations, for complex social systems can be understood only through an analysis of the actions of their subparts and an analysis of the interactions between these subparts. Hospitals, other health-care organizations, and institutions of higher education are complex social systems with personnel, clients, and services that constantly act and interact. A health-care consortium is even more complex. Design provides a way of finding solutions and consists of cycles of imaging, presenting, testing, critical reflection, and reimaging. Participants in interactive planning processes share their own particular visions and discover common themes. In this way, members of the system develop a shared image and understanding. Testing is then done through taking action, reflecting, critiquing action, evaluating, and refining or re-creating the design as needed.

The experience Health Bond service and education participants had in cross-discipline and cross-organization interactive planning teams influenced their conceptualization of ways to meet identified community needs through community-based, nurse-managed interdisciplinary care innovations, and their creation of novel service-learning curricula options for their students. The senior citizen health clinic is a remarkable example of this kind of development.

Consumer-Centered Services

Positive experiences with the interdisciplinary hospice model influenced the readiness of Health Bond participants to learn and apply an interactive planning process. The central position of the patient and family, clergy, and lay volunteers on a team that includes an interdisciplinary mix of providers representing community care and long-term care and acute care was critical to the selection of this model as the template for all patient care and consumer health services in the Health Bond Consortium. A variety of innovations related to health-care services, including interregional case management, have been developed through the Health Bond Consortium. These innovations address the client's continuum of care and create new opportunities and settings for interdisciplinary service-learning in the community (Aadalen et al. 1996; McBeth and Weydt 1996).

Shared Governance Structure for Service/Education Partnership Development

Shared governance is a decentralized structure for decision making at a departmental, organizational, interorganizational, regional, and/or state level. When the Health Bond Consortium initially formed to develop a planning grant proposal (1989-1990), there was little to no information in the literature about shared governance other than at the departmental level (Porter-O'Grady and Finnigan 1984). Movement beyond this level was evident in an early 1990s publication related to creating a professional organization (Porter-O'Grady 1992).

The Health Bond Consortium designed an interorganizational shared governance structure to manage decision making and the grant budget, to promote leadership development, to provide internal consultation for innovation teams related to regional initiatives, to promote coordinated action toward achievement of project objectives and progress toward the shared vision, and to define responsibility, authority, and accountability for the action research evaluation. This shared governance structure had a coordinating council and executive committee and four standing committees: regional health-care advisory; quality, evaluation, and research; decentralized patient-care delivery systems; and education and information. This structure is like a hologram: Each part is representative of the whole, having representatives from education and patient services, the community, health-care consumers, and major provider groups. The shared governance structure thus supported service and education partnership development through its structure and processes and as a valued outcome (McBeth et al. 1995).

Shared Learning Experiences

Developing trust in service and education partnerships has been facilitated by shared learning experiences that focused on effective, responsible communication, effective relationship management, leadership development in self and others, care-delivery system innovations, and collaborative decision making. To begin with, the shared learning was across departmental and discipline lines within an organization (hospital), a school, or division (higher education), and focused on developing the leadership skills that facilitate the development of others. Administrators (service and education), middle managers, faculty, and lead workers all had the opportunity and were encouraged to participate in communication strengthening, relationship building, and leadership development experiential education.

Subsequent consultation and education sessions had participants representing two rural hospitals, a regional health center, a technical college, and the state university. The experiential and team learning nature of these learning retreats opened participant perspectives to new visions of the possible. They were extremely important in helping them to move from the paradigm of an episodic illness–care system within the walls not only of a hospital but also of a particular unit or department, to a paradigm of integrated health and education systems — new partnerships collaborating to meet the needs of the individual and family life-health continuums and beyond to the health of the community.

Clinical and internship learning experiences for university and technical students from a variety of disciplines at the regional health center and rural primary-care hospitals changed because the faculty and organizational staff had the opportunity to participate in shared learning experiences together. They shared a language and meaning system that included the commitment to empowering staff and students, and clear articulation of levels of responsibility, authority, and accountability. Most of all, the covert curricula became very clear: Education and service providers who partner together, maximizing limited expertise and other resources, can co-evolve, with their staff and students, significant service-learning opportunities. Diverse individuals become bonded in a cause greater than themselves.

Learning Organization Disciplines

People are the most valuable resources available. In a world of extraordinary change, with the pace of change increasing logarithmically, organizations whose employees are willing and eager to work together to learn new and better approaches to omnipresent challenges reap many benefits from a committed, flexible, adaptable workforce.

Administrators in Health Bond organizations made a commitment to employee education and development. Shared study of Peter Senge's book

The Fifth Discipline: The Art and Practice of the Learning Organization (1990) allowed executive administrators, managers and directors, faculty, and grass-roots staff to learn about, practice, and have an opportunity to integrate new behaviors related to his five core disciplines of learning organizations. These disciplines are personal mastery, critique and reflect mental models, shared visioning, team learning, and systems thinking.

Health Bond created the opportunity for interdisciplinary service/education innovation project teams to form and develop proposals for small-grant funding to carry out projects that were regional in scope. Twenty-eight innovation projects were implemented (Health Bond 1994). Examples include Maternal Child Services Integration, Better Communication With Sexual Assault Victims and Survivors, Hospice: Meeting the Needs of Patients and Families, Interregional Collaborative Cardiovascular Project (Heart Health Care Notebook), Dysphagia Project, Oncology Resources Project, and Faith-Health Ministry. Each of the 28 projects provided mastery learning opportunities related to Peter Senge's five disciplines.

Action-Oriented Evaluation

Health Bond's vision of continuous improvement in the quality, cost-effectiveness, responsiveness, and coordination of health-care services in south central Minnesota mandated an action research approach to evaluation of initiatives. While Health Bond initiated and implemented change, the consortium governance bodies studied the processes underlying innovations, evaluated them, and continually learned from them (Health Bond 1995).

Service-Learning: Linkage and Practice Issues

Developing ongoing service and education partnership dialogue about health-care practice programs and education curricula facilitates building service-learning opportunities. Challenges to this change toward greater service/education curriculum integration for the community's health include (1) accreditation requirements that may lag behind changing demands of the practice workplace arena, (2) limited funding to support the development of service-learning opportunities, (3) the time and energy required to establish and implement innovative service-learning initiatives, (4) institutional reward systems based on linear, hierarchical, individualistic orientations, and (5) a dearth of institutionalized mechanisms to free staff and faculty over time for participation in innovative service-learning initiatives. The Health Bond service/education partnership consortium demonstrates how to meet these challenges through collaborative relationships with community partners, which are nurtured and sustained over time.

Clearly, the costs of higher education and health care must be contained while providing quality education/services that yield demonstrable positive outcomes. Sharing resources across traditional departmental and institutional boundaries through the formation of meaningful, informal community relationships is one key strategy. The structured integration of community service experiences with academic and employment objectives is a powerful mechanism for resource sharing and service/education quality. Ideally, students receive credit for team learning experiences in which faculty, staff, students, and clients are engaged in service-learning experiences together rather than for hours of service. Adequate preparation of students for the service-learning experience and evaluation of student, staff, professional colleague, and community outcomes must be continuous, vigorous, and coordinated. When service-learning is implemented in this way, strong academic performance, the development of caring compassion, and civic responsibility are predictable outcomes for lifelong learners in nursing.

Note

1. An example is the Minnesota Campus Compact, a coalition of 45 college and university presidents that encourages student involvement in community and public service, and strengthens the impact of that service on the welfare of communities and the education of students in Minnesota (Langseth 1996).

References

Aadalen, S., C. Ahern, D. Schiro, T. Thomas, and A. Weydt. (1996). "A 12-Month Post-Acute Care Clinical Path: Implications for Home Care Nursing." In *Home Care & Clinical Paths: Effective Care Planning Across the Continuum,* edited by T.M. Marrelli and L.S. Hilliard, 189-200. St. Louis, MO: Mosby Yearbook.

Aadalen, S., A. McBeth, L. Froehlich, M.K. Hohenstein, S. Raetz, and K. Schweer. (1997). "Transforming Healthcare Systems." In *The Executive Nurse: Leadership for New Health Care Transitions,* edited by Sandera R. Byers, Chap. 6. Albany, NY: Delmar.

Ackoff, R.L. (February 1989). "The Circular Organization: An Update." *Academy of Management Executives* 3(1): 11-16.

Ashley, J. (1976). *Hospitals, Paternalism, and the Role of the Nurse.* New York, NY: Teachers College Press.

Boyer, E.L. (1990). *Scholarship Reconsidered: Priorities of the Professoriate.* Princeton, NJ: Carnegie Foundation for the Advancement of Teaching.

Greater New York Hospital Association. (1996). *Project L.I.N.C.: The Ladders in Nursing Careers Program: Building Bridges.* New York, NY: Greater New York Hospital Association.

Health Bond. (Winter/Spring 1994). *Newsletter* 4(1).

——— . (October 1995). *Strengthening Hospital Nursing Program Final Evaluation Report.* Mankato, MN: Health Bond.

Johnson, M., and M. Maas, eds. (1997). *Nursing Outcomes Classification (NOC).* St. Louis, MO: Mosby Yearbook.

Langseth, M. (Winter 1996). "From Shakespeare to Chemistry: A Guide to Service-Learning." *Faculty Development: The Collaboration for the Advancement of College Teaching and Learning* 9(2): 1-2.

McBeth, A., K. Schweer, and S. Aadalen. (1995). "Health Bond." In *Transformational Leadership: Renewing Fundamental Values and Achieving New Relationships in Health Care,* edited by M.K. Kohles, W.G. Baker, and B.A. Donaho, Chap. 12. Chicago, IL: American Hospital Publishing Co.

McBeth, A., and A. Weydt. (1996). "Innovative Delivery Systems, Freedom, Trust, and Caring." In *Nurse Case Management in the 21st Century,* edited by E. Cohen, Chap. 12. St. Louis, MO: Mosby Yearbook.

McCloskey, J.C., and G.M. Bulecheck, eds. (1996). *Nursing Interventions Classification (NIC).* St. Louis, MO: Mosby Yearbook.

National Commission on Nursing Implementation Project. (May 1, 1990). *NCNIP Report to the W.K. Kellogg Foundation. Year Five.* Milwaukee, WI: National Commission on Nursing Implementation Project.

North American Nursing Diagnosis Association. (1996). *NANDA Nursing Diagnosis: Definitions and Classifications, 1997-1998.* Philadelphia, PA: North American Nursing Diagnosis Association.

Palmer, P. (November 1995). "The Renewal of Community in Higher Education." Keynote address at the Opening the Classroom Door: Fostering Learning, Strengthening Community conference of the Collaboration for the Advancement of College Teaching and Learning, St. Paul, MN.

Porter-O'Grady, T. (1992). *Implementing Shared Governance: Creating a Professional Organization.* St. Louis, MO: Mosby Yearbook.

——— , and S. Finnigan. (1984). *Shared Governance for Nursing: A Creative Approach to Professional Accountability.* Gaithersburg, MD: Aspen.

Rush, S.L. (1992). "Nursing Education in the United States, 1898-1910: A Time of Auspicious Beginnings." *Journal of Nursing Education* 31(9): 409-414.

Rydholm, L. (1997). "Patient-Focused Care in Parish Nursing." *Holistic Nursing Practice* 11(3): 47-60.

Senge, P.M. (1990). *The Fifth Discipline: The Art and Practice of the Learning Organization.* New York, NY: Doubleday Currency.

Strengthening Hospital Nursing: A Program to Improve Patient Care. (Spring 1992-Winter 1995). *Strengthening,* vol. 1, nos. 1-4.

Teagle Foundation. (1996). *LPN-to-BSN Initiative*. New York, NY: Teagle Foundation.

Service-Learning as a Pedagogy in Nursing

by Elaine Cohen, Susan Johnson, Lois Nelson, and Connie Peterson

The profession of nursing is currently surrounded by and immersed in a whirlwind of change in the health-care delivery system. Prospective payment strategies, redefinition of the client as consumer, corporatization of hospitals, downsizing, and sweeping technological changes have all become critical issues that need to be addressed in the practice arena. All of these factors have increased the level of difficulty in preparing a professional nurse to be an effective practitioner. How do educational institutions sensitize students to the challenges being faced by clients who are of multiple cultural and socioeconomic groups? How can educational institutions continue to provide quality clinical experiences when their own downsizing jeopardizes the traditional view of how clinical experiences are supervised? How can students be prepared to think independently and be provided with opportunities to develop their skill in self-direction? How can the institution prepare students to practice in nursing settings that have not yet been well defined in the current health-care system? How can students learn about possible gaps in the continuum of care so that they can begin to sense future nursing opportunities? A partial answer to these questions may be found in the concept of service-learning, a concept that arises from the historical roots of the profession of nursing. It has been said that answers to the future may lie in the past. This may very well be true in the profession of nursing.

Historical Perspectives

The concept of community service dates back to the time of the ancient Hebrews, when nurses participated in visiting the sick and supporting the family care givers with food and spiritual refreshment. During this period of history, and many hundreds of years later, there was a strong religious component to the practice of nursing. Secular nursing orders also arose during this time, providing voluntary services and care during several of the famines and epidemics of the era (Dolan 1978).

The modern era of nursing had its roots in the 1850s with the teachings of Florence Nightingale. Her book, *Notes on Nursing* (London: Harrison & Sons, 1859), was to become one of the defining texts on the practice of nursing. She was one of the first to formally identify two major components of nursing — health nursing and sick nursing — and she was a strong proponent for primary prevention and health maintenance.

As the history of professional nursing is analyzed, the concepts of service, vocation, and community health are recurrent themes. How can this message be translated into current practice? The following case study on incorporating a service-learning project into the nursing curriculum in the college setting is one attempt to provide an answer.

Initiation of a Service-Learning Project

Educational Goals

The purpose of integrating a service-learning clinical component into the nursing curriculum was to provide timely experiences whereby students could apply theoretical content to actual nursing settings. The service-learning experience was designed to address several broad curricular goals. These goals include integrating the concept of nursing in the community setting across the nursing major, broadening the perception of the role of the nurse in society, strengthening communication skills, and fostering the development of autonomy and self-directed learning skills. Integration of a service-learning project was also an attempt to provide students the opportunity to further develop as responsible and effective citizens in the context of professional nursing. This particular goal is congruent with the mission statement of the nursing program, which states that "the mission of the nursing program is to promote health by preparing professional nurses and serving as a nursing resource to society."

With these objectives in mind, faculty incorporated a service-learning experience into a second-semester junior-level course entitled Nursing Concepts (see Set 1 in the "Samples" section of this volume). This course was perceived by faculty as being especially appropriate for a service-learning clinical component because of the topics addressed. These topics included spiritual health, sociocultural perspectives in nursing, death and dying, health promotion for clients with a chronic illness, substance abuse, and some common disorders in the adult population. The selection of service-learning sites was based on relevance to these course topics. The following sites were contacted for student placement: a hospice, churches with parish nursing programs, a diabetic screening program, a refugee resettlement program, retirement centers, homeless shelters, and an Indian health center. The concept map *opposite* correlates the primary course concepts with the service-learning sites and relevant nursing skills utilized by students.

Agency Coordination

It was important to share the concept of service-learning with participating agencies, determine the number of hours required for project completion (20 hours), identify the number of students the agency could accommodate, and identify activities the students were able to perform appropri-

Service-Learning Concept Map

Service-Learning Site	Course Concepts	Primary Skills Applied
Hospice	death and dying, spirituality	communication, assessment
Parish nursing programs	spirituality, chronic illness, parish nurse role	assessment, communication, client education
Diabetic screening	chronic illness, sensory disorders, integumentary disorders	assessment, communication, client education
Lutheran Social Services refugee resettlement program	sociocultural perspectives	communication, client education, critical thinking
Retirement center	sociocultural perspectives, chronic illness, sensory and mobility disorders	communication, assessment
Community health centers (homeless shelters, Indian health center)	sociocultural perspectives, substance abuse	assessment, communication, client teaching

ate for the purposes of this project. Orientation was mutually arranged between the students and the agencies. Each student provided the agency with a learning agreement form (reproduced at the end of this chapter) identifying the service expectations.

Designing Student Assignments

A vital aspect of this project was to design assignments to enable students to reflect critically on their service-learning experience and to link their experiences to course material (see Set 1 in the "Samples" section of this volume for the assignment sheet). The assignment encouraged personal reflection and critical thinking. There were three written assignments that served the broader college writing goal of developing written communication skills. The first paper was entitled "Preparation for Service-Learning." The purpose of this paper was for the student to investigate the role of the agency as a community resource. It was designed to have the students explore current research findings in preparation for service-learning participation.

The second assignment required students to write periodically in a journal. In the journals, they listed date and hours worked, a description of what service activities were performed, a discussion of how the experience was linked to course content, and a reflection on the student's own personal role development. Comments included personal reactions and knowledge and skills acquired or reinforced.

The third written assignment was a final report on the service-learning project (see Set 1 for a sample report). After completing the service-learning project, students were to answer the following questions in the report: How did the experience relate to the course topics? What knowledge and skills were gained? How did it expand on your thoughts about nursing? How could you have done things differently to gain more from the experience?

The students were assigned to groups to present highlights of significant learning experiences to their classmates. In this way, other students became aware of all the community resources utilized in this project. No matter where these students practice in the future, it will be vital for them to be knowledgeable about many resources that may be available to clients. This class sharing was an important part of the learning experience, because knowledge of community resources is essential for effective nursing practice in the complex health-care environment.

Implementation: One Example

Diabetic Screening Project

The service-learning site that had the greatest number of students was the North Dakota State Diabetes Screening Program. This site will be highlighted as an example of the service-learning project.

The diabetic screening project was directed by a certified diabetic educator at the Dakota Heartland Health System. The target population was diabetic clients in the community. The rate of diabetes in North Dakota is of concern because it is twice the rate of the general population in the United States and because complications of diabetes cause considerable morbidity and increased economic costs. This screening was developed to identify diabetic complications at an early stage, as well as to teach preventative care. It also provided an opportunity to collect data about diabetes for future programming.

The screening program consisted of nine separate stations where clients were assessed for current health status and their knowledge about diabetes. In order to staff these stations, volunteers were needed. Thus, it was an ideal situation for students who needed placement for a service-learning project. The stations in which the students participated included admitting/history, height and weight, blood pressure, blood glucose, visual acuity, and foot examination. The faculty worked with the agency personnel to facilitate orientation and distribution of educational materials for the preparation of students. The students were expected to prepare themselves and assist in setting up the site for the screening activities. The students rotated working at the various stations at subsequent screenings so they could learn different skills.

Student Reflections

Communicating with clients in this type of setting was a new learning experience for the students. They were confronted with the challenge of establishing rapport with clients within a short time period. They gained skill in admitting clients, orienting them to a new setting, and teaching health information in a non-acute-care setting.

The students broadened their understanding of diabetes management and complications such as visual problems and hypertension. They were able to grasp what it means to people to have a chronic illness, how it affects their lives, and how it requires many life-style changes. They discovered how individual clients vary in their response to diabetes. For example, some clients followed their diabetic diets and medication almost obsessively, while others were very noncompliant with their diabetic regimes.

Students remarked about how they enjoyed the teamwork involved in implementation of this screening project. It was offered three times, which helped develop a sense of community among the students as they cooperated in accomplishing a common goal. They appreciated being exposed to a special nursing role, the diabetic nurse-educator. They appreciated the benefits of a free screening service for clients, many of whom do not regularly see a health-care provider. Some of the clients remarked that they had never been so thoroughly evaluated, especially with the foot examination. Thus, the students were conscious of the fact that they were providing a comprehensive and high-quality program. This was beneficial for their self-confidence, knowing they had knowledge and skills that they could share with clients. Students could perceive how this type of service might be useful in other arenas of health care. They also gained a view of health care as being more of a partnership with the client.

Agency Reflections

The clinical agency perceived student participation as a significant factor in the success of the diabetic screening program. The project was very labor-intensive and students provided vital manpower, as each station required an examination and client education. The screening was a way for the participants to have contact with a nonphysician health-care provider who could be a resource for their future diabetic management. From the agency's perspective, the students and community gained an awareness of the agency's commitment to prevention and treatment of diabetes. An added benefit to the agency was the influence of the screening project on the potential recruitment of graduates.

Project Evaluation

Evaluation of the service-learning experience was an inherent part of the design of the course. Students were surveyed immediately following the conclusion of the course and again after one year concerning their response to the project. The areas of professional role development are displayed in the table *opposite*.

The highest-ranking item was communication skills, followed by appreciation of the value of community service and gaining confidence in their abilities. Although experience with writing skills and learning about a culture/class different from their own were ranked eighth and ninth, the mean evaluation was still high, 3.6.

Students were also given the opportunity to comment on the experience. The most frequent comments concerned the importance of improving communication skills as well as communicating with those from other cultures, especially those speaking limited English. Next in frequency were comments related to the importance of client education/health promotion, and third was the importance of spirituality in nursing.

In the one-year postproject evaluation, the students were again requested to respond to a survey asking them how they perceived their attainment

Immediate Postproject Student Evaluation

Rank	Areas of Development	Mean
1	Experience with oral communicationskills	4.66
2	Appreciate the value of communityservice	4.50
3	Gain confidence in your abilities	4.43
4	Apply course content to the real world	4.30
5	Consider different roles for nursing	4.29
6	Critically reflect on your values and biases	4.08
7	Experience with problem solving, critical thinking	3.88
8	Experience with writing skills	3.60
9	Learn about a culture/class different from your own	3.56

Note: n = 47. The rating was on a five-point scale, with 5="strongly agree" and 1="strongly disagree."

of the course objectives relating to service-learning. The results of this evaluation are provided in the table *opposite*. The objective that was perceived as being met by the highest number of students (78.7%) was "Appreciate the potential roles of nursing in the community setting." This perspective remained high in importance even after one year after the project completion. The two objectives having the lowest ranking (7 and 8) were "Gain insight into potential areas of employment in my future nursing career" and "Gain insight into the value system of someone from a culture different from my own." Even though they had the lowest ranking, 46.8 percent of the students perceived they met objective 7, and 38.3 percent met objective 8. A possible explanation for the lower ranking might be the nature of the service-learning site to which the student was assigned. For example, in the refugee resettlement program learning experience, cultural differences were a primary focus. In the hospice experience, however, spiritual and communication issues were most important.

Faculty response to the service-learning experience was very positive. They were pleased to note that the students' evaluations reflected the broad curricular goals utilized in designing the project as well as achievement of specific course theory objectives. The senior-level faculty reported that students who had completed the service-learning clinical component were more sensitized to the role of the nurse in the community setting. They were also more knowledgeable about community health resources and more comfortable with interdisciplinary communication. The faculty also noted that the item scored the second highest by students evaluating the service-learning experience was that of appreciating the value of community service as a part of citizenship. This feedback reinforced the service mission of the nursing program.

Challenges

In the implementation of a course project with many students in different areas, problems will arise. Students need to be encouraged to approach the problems with a sense of creativity, initiative, and self-direction. While the diabetic screening program was quite directive in what students would be doing, other sites demanded more initiative on the students' part to make them a quality learning experience. For example, it would be easy for students involved in parish nursing to just take blood pressures during a blood pressure screening period at the church. The learning and serving would be present, but the learning would be limited in scope. Therefore, it was necessary to give the students some ideas and approaches with their site supervisor to expand on their service experience. For example, students assisted in planning and implementing health fairs, wrote an article focused on

Student Perceptions: One-Year Postproject Evaluation

Rank	Objective	Met Percentage (Number)	Partially Met Percentage (Number)	Not Met Percentage (Number)
1	Appreciate the potential roles of nursing in the community setting in order to serve as a nursing resource for society.	78.7 (37)	17.0 (8)	4.3 (2)
2	Appreciate the inherent values and benefits of service as part of effective citizenship.	76.6 (36)	21.3 (10)	2.1 (1)
3	Gain familiarity with health resources available in the community setting.	63.8 (30)	31.9 (15)	4.3 (2)
4	Gain insight into my own value system.	63.8 (30)	34.0 (16)	2.1 (1)
5	Gain confidence in the development of my own professional nursing role.	57.4 (27)	36.2 (17)	6.4 (3)
6	Apply new course content as well as previous learning to clients outside the acute-care setting.	55.3 (26)	36.2 (17)	8.5 (4)
7	Gain insight into potential areas of employment in my future nursing career.	46.8 (22)	38.3 (18)	14.9 (7)
8	Gain insight into the value system of someone from a culture different from my own.	38.3 (18)	40.4 (19)	21.3 (10)

Note: n = 47

health for the church newsletter, or did research on community resources for the parish nurse program.

Other challenges that occurred were changes in personnel. In some instances, when the student contacted the agency as instructed there was a different person in the position, who may or may not have understood the philosophy of service-learning and what arrangements had previously been made. Such glitches required more phone calls and time for the faculty, and left students feeling somewhat bewildered.

Nursing curricula demand heavy commitments of time and study. The students have limited time outside of class and laboratory to coordinate their service-learning contract. Occasionally bad weather conditions prompted cancellations, and rescheduling was a source of frustration and a problem for students.

From the faculty perspective, it is more manageable to keep the number of project sites to a minimum. However, achieving this goal depends most directly on the number of students in the class and the number of students each agency is able to accommodate. It is extremely helpful if the faculty member is knowledgeable about the agency and has a good working relationship with the staff. This takes time, and supports the guideline of limiting the number of agencies involved.

Conclusions

The concept of service is deeply rooted in the nursing profession. This project was a natural outgrowth of this rich history. Faculty, students, and agencies involved with the implementation of this project benefited from their involvement. Students spoke of applying course content in "real life" and "learning things they could not have learned in the classroom." They also stated that they had gained cultural awareness, communication skills, familiarity with other nursing roles, and organizational skills. A few students opted to continue their service activities as a direct result of the project. Faculty and agency personnel gained a new perspective on working collaboratively to pursue mutual goals. Faculty increased their comfort level with serving as consultants rather than as direct supervisors of student activities.

The success of this project makes it a viable addition to more traditional clinical practicum experiences. Service-learning is one way to address the difficult challenges facing nursing education today.

Reference

Dolan, J.A. (1978). *Nursing in Society: A Historical Perspective*. Philadelphia, PA: W.B. Saunders.

Tri-College University Nursing Consortium/
Concordia College and North Dakota State University

Student Service-Learning Project Agreement

This agreement is for the purpose of clarifying service activities, number of hours, and accountabilities of the nursing student for the service-learning project in Nursing 351, Nursing Concepts.

As a participant, the STUDENT agrees to the following:

1. Serve a minimum of 20 hours over the course of the semester. The agency will be contacted ahead of time in case of absences that occur due to emergencies and illness.

2. Attend meetings that are deemed necessary by the agency served, unless there are class conflicts.

3. Provide a record of service hours to the site supervisor on an ongoing basis. (If special prep time is needed, these hours are counted.)

4. Respect the rules and regulations, including all confidences of the agency and clients being served.

5. Follow professional guidelines expected of students during the clinical practicum.

6. Perform the following activities listed below.

_____   _____
(Student Signature)   (Date)

The following service activities will be performed by the student:

Name of Agency:_____

I agree to the above service activities:

_____   _____
(Supervisor/Contact Person for Student)   (Date)

Copy to agency and course instructor, Susan Johnson, assistant professor of nursing at Concordia College, ph 299-4063.

Case Study of a Service-Learning Project in a Nurse-Managed Clinic for Homeless and Indigent Individuals

by Carol L. Macnee, Deborah H. White, and Jean C. Hemphill

This chapter describes the implementation of two service-learning courses within the setting of a primary-care clinic for homeless and indigent individuals. The two courses are a campus-wide Introduction to Community Service and a Community Health Nursing Practicum. Although these two courses have different learning outcomes, they both address the primary goals of service-learning, including (1) developing students' understanding about the responsibility of citizenship and preparing students for effective roles in society; (2) improving students' communication skills, problem-solving skills, and project-specific skills; (3) enhancing students' self-esteem and sense of social reality; and (4) providing an interdisciplinary perspective (Kendall and Associates 1990). The sections that follow describe the setting that the two service-learning courses share, the university-wide course, and the community health nursing practicum. Common issues faced in both courses that are discussed include reflective learning practices, community/client impact, communicating expectations to the student and the site personnel, collaboration to accomplish both service and learning outcomes, and practical issues associated with service-learning in a clinic for the homeless and indigent.

The Setting for the Service-Learning Courses

The Johnson City Downtown Clinic for Homeless (JCDTC) is the setting shared by both service-learning courses described in this chapter. JCDTC is a nurse-managed primary-care clinic that provides advanced nursing care in collaboration with a medical preceptor to homeless and indigent people without charge. In addition to traditional management of acute and chronic physical and mental health problems, the clinic provides a safe, supportive environment for socializing; assistance with acquisition of medications and referrals; screening for health problems such as hypertension, diabetes,

---

Support provided by a Special Projects Grant from the Division of Nursing, Bureau of Health Professions, Health and Human Services Grant 1 D10 NU30187-01.

or foot problems; health education and promotion; personal hygiene supplies and assistance with acquiring food and shelter; and outreach to local housing projects, shelters for the homeless, and the streets for case finding and screening.

The JCDTC is jointly sponsored by the East Tennessee State University College of Nursing and the City of Johnson City and is supported by local, state, and federal grants, donations, and some third-party reimbursement. Staff in the clinic include full-time family nurse practitioners, a psychiatric clinical nurse specialist two days per week, one full-time baccalaureate-prepared nurse, and a secretary/receptionist. The clinic is open four days a week and provides care to clients on a first-come, first-served basis, with ill children given priority. Due to space and staff limitations, clients often have as long as an hour wait before being seen in the clinic, and currently there are an average of 400 client encounters each month in the clinic.

The clinic provides care in an open and relatively unstructured manner, which allows clients the freedom to come and go from the clinic as needed for reasons ranging from a job interview, the lunch meal program opening, or the need to smoke a cigarette outside. It is not necessary to be seeking traditional primary health care to come to the clinic or to be seen. Management of acute and chronic health problems does not usually begin until 9:00 am; however, the nurse opens the clinic doors early each morning to allow potential clients to use the waiting area for rest, security, and socialization, and to get a free cup of coffee.

The Campus-Wide Course: Introduction to Service-Learning

The Introduction to Service-Learning course gives students an interdisciplinary look at community issues such as health care, hunger and homelessness, education, and public safety. It explores the role of leadership in efforts of change and supports students' efforts to assume those roles. Students spend 30 to 40 hours in a service placement and two to three hours per week in class engaged in reflective learning activities, and they write about their experiences and research the issues surrounding their particular placement. Although the course is open to any student in the university, generally it has been third- and fourth-year students who have enrolled in the course. Twelve nursing majors elected to take this course in its first year.

Through the Office of Student Activities, East Tennessee State University developed a vision for a campus-wide service-learning course in 1994. Using the success of the campus elective center as a springboard, the Introduction course was piloted in spring 1995 in cooperation with the Department of Human Development and Learning in the College of Education. It was funded by the Corporation for National Service with a grant from Learn and

Serve America. Other colleges on campus soon gave their support to the course and to the entire service-learning effort.

The Introduction course (see Set 2 in the "Samples" section of this volume for the syllabus) begins with an overview of community needs through a variety of guest speakers from agencies in a six-county region of northeastern Tennessee. All students gain a level of understanding regarding the range of community needs and will discover the interrelation of these needs as the course progresses. The students select an area of interest in which they would like to serve, and they review agency project descriptions. After consultation with the program site placement coordinator, the student is placed in an agency for a 30-hour service placement to be completed by the end of the semester. The classwork during this time includes a short research paper on the issue/agency in which they are working, several reflective learning experiences through group presentations and journals, and simulation games on issues of diversity and homelessness. Lappé and Du Bois's book *The Quickening of America* (Jossey-Bass, 1994) serves as the text. Concepts of social justice, leadership for social change, and a multicultural society are explored.

Group Service Project

As part of the course, students are required to participate in a group service project with service-learning students from other nearby campuses. This knowledge of the emphasis on service of many campuses around the region, state, and country is important to the students' perspective about service as a lifelong commitment. Another important segment of the class that serves as an individual reflection tool and a personal development model is the leadership transcript exercise. This session provides an in-depth look at one's strengths and how service-learning experiences are steps in a process of personal leadership development. Students are offered the opportunity to set up an actual cocurricular transcript record that they can update and access throughout their college career. Through this emphasis on service as a lifetime commitment, 30 percent of students are remaining with their service placements after the class is completed. Another 20 percent have sought a second placement. Because the Introduction course had been offered for only three semesters at the time this chapter was written, a longitudinal follow-up has not yet been possible.

To date, service activities of students from the campus-wide Introduction course who have participated in the JCDTC program have included assisting with sign-in and record keeping in the clinic, provision of social support to clients in the waiting/reception area, and assistance with sorting and organizing donations to the clinic, including clothes, food, and medicines. Other nursing student placements have included health education roles in after-school programs and patient support services in area hospitals and rural clinics.

Finding suitable service-learning placements in health care can be difficult without careful planning. Prior to the semester offering the service-learning course, the site placement coordinator seeks to communicate with the agency representatives who will supervise the student placements. Annually, an agency training session is held to orient these participant coordinators about the best ways to use a service-learning student. These interactions help define the concept of service-learning for the agencies, conceptualize project descriptions for student learning, and relay the expectations of the course instructor regarding student training and evaluation within the total course evaluations. Specific to health-care placements, concerns of safety and liability, immunizations, screening of students, and training for medical protocols are issues that must be addressed to the satisfaction of the health-care agencies. All such agreements and processes are best put into writing and reviewed by the university's general counsel. This requires cooperation and collaboration between the support personnel for the course, the health-care agency, and the College of Nursing faculty.

Before the students are placed in an agency, part of a class session is devoted to expectations of the students at their sites. This includes such topics as attendance, attire, punctuality, and other professional behaviors. Many agencies, especially health-care agencies, will check police records and require health screenings and immunizations. Students placed in direct health-care delivery services must meet all OSHA criteria, including TB testing, opportunity for a Hepatitis B vaccination, and documentation of a rubella titer or MMR. Prior arrangements with the local health department or campus health center can provide such screenings and services to students at low or no cost.

Ongoing site supervision is handled through the agency supervisor and the site placement coordinator. Ongoing evaluation is found in the students' reflection journals. Student and agency focus groups are held annually to assess any needed changes. Formal written evaluations are completed in various ways: by the students about the faculty member, by agencies about the students, and by the students about the agencies. To reduce issues of liability, students sign a "hold harmless" agreement and must provide their own transportation to the agency. Agencies must also sign an agreement to provide a positive educational work environment for the student.

The Community Health Nursing Practicum

Part of the vision for service-learning at East Tennessee State University is to infuse such opportunities across the curriculum into preexisting classes.

The College of Nursing was one of the first at ETSU to offer a course with a service-learning component. The Community Health Nursing Practicum (see Set 2 for its syllabus) is a five-credit clinical course that is open only to senior baccalaureate nursing students. The content emphasizes providing population-focused and culturally relevant care focused on health promotion and disease prevention to individuals, families, and groups in home and community settings. Opportunities for student experiences in the roles of case finder, care provider, service coordinator, collaborator, consultant, advocate, and health program planner are sought. Learning outcomes of the course include (1) implementing strategies designed to promote the health of individuals, families, and selected populations at risk by using the nursing process, critical-thinking/diagnostic reasoning skills, and therapeutic communication; (2) working in partnership with clients in the context of cultural and individual differences when planning, implementing, and evaluating community health nursing care; (3) collaborating with other professionals when providing community health nursing care; and (4) using pertinent community resources that are consistent with clients' health-care needs.

Students spend approximately 55 hours in clinical settings and approximately six hours per week in small groups. The small-group work includes an aggregate-focused project, a written clinical critique, and seminar/conferences regarding their clinical experiences. Clinical settings for students include traditional public health departments, school-based clinics, and the JCDTC. Approximately 18 to 20 nursing students (33% of the course enrollment) participate in delivering services at the JCDTC each semester.

While service-learning is a potential teaching method in any of the clinical settings used in this Community Health Nursing Practicum, the JCDTC was established and developed with service-learning as one of the major goals. The clinic represents a partnership between the City of Johnson City and the College of Nursing for the specific purposes of providing service to homeless and indigent individuals and providing academic learning opportunities with underserved populations for nursing students.

Because the JCDTC was established with an expectation that service-learning would occur, collaboration to accomplish both service and learning outcomes has not been as difficult as it might be in other settings. However, the clinic faces the daily challenge of meeting many complex health needs within the context of limited space, staff, and resources. Initially, learning experiences in the clinic for undergraduate students were limited to a one-day experience for one or two students. When it was decided to place a clinical section of students at the JCDTC, the clinic staff were excited about the opportunity for more students to learn within their unique care setting, but they were also concerned about the effect more students might have on their ability to provide care. The introduction of at least five or six students who would physically occupy some of the very limited space, who were not familiar with clinic routine, and who were in the process of learning their roles had the potential to disrupt the flow of clinic services and therefore negatively impact service outcomes. At the same time, course faculty were concerned that the space and resource limitations of the clinic might limit opportunities for students to actively learn and participate in the delivery of care.

Screening Programs

These concerns regarding accomplishing both service and learning outcomes were resolved collaboratively by identifying two major activities for student learning. The first major service-learning activity in the JCDTC was the provision of weekly screening programs for diabetes, hypertension, anemia, and foot problems. These screening programs are offered only during the weeks that students are in the clinic; therefore, they reflect a direct and unique service to the community. At the same time, the screening clinics provide opportunities for the students to accomplish many of the outcomes for the Community Health Nursing Practicum. Concerns about limited space are in part resolved by these screening programs, because the students, under supervision of College of Nursing faculty, set up and implement a screening clinic each week in an anteroom set off from the JCDTC itself.

The screening clinics are advertised each week through flyers posted at the local shelters, in the dining area for the daily meal program, and in the clinic itself. Clients are invited to receive screening independent of whether they use regular clinic services. Screenings include brief histories to assess for risk factors and significant health history related to the problem being screened, followed by the screening procedure itself and then counseling regarding need for follow-up and appropriate self-care. Students implement all aspects of the screenings, from setting up the equipment and area to filing completed screening forms on charts of individuals who have charts in the regular clinic (Macnee et al. 1996).

Provision of Care

The second major service-learning activity in the JCDTC is rotation of two students at a time into the regular JCDTC to assist in the provision of all aspects of care that are routinely provided in the clinic. As students finish working with a client within the clinic itself, they come back out to the screening clinic, allowing another student to pick up and work with a client within the regular clinic. Rather than disrupting clinical services as feared, this approach to student participation in the clinic has meant that it is often possible to provide care to more clients than would receive care with regular staffing of the clinic. In particular, students provide labor-intensive care such as detailed diabetic teaching or support and assistance in special referral services, which sometimes are not possible for regular staff to provide. The care provided by students in the clinic accomplishes course outcomes for academic learning about community health nursing while providing important services to the homeless and indigent clients seen in the clinic.

Practical Issues

Practical issues that have needed to be worked out for this service-learning experience have included management of student flow in and out of the clinic, extent of student participation in client documentation, and details such as student parking and storing of coats and purses. Clinic staff were particularly concerned that continuity of care be maintained when students were participating in client care. Therefore, the baccalaureate-prepared nurse in the clinic has accepted the role of "director" of student/client assignments, while faculty are responsible for assuring that students participate in both the screening and the regular clinic and have specific, individually identified learning opportunities. It was agreed that once a student worked with a particular client, the same student would continue to follow that client throughout his or her clinic visit. However, when a particular client is waiting for results of tests or to be taken to an exam room, the student may be asked to assist with some other aspect of clinic services. Thus, students, faculty, and staff work collaboratively to provide flexible and fluid services that meet both learning and health-care outcomes.

Other practical issues were resolved by agreeing that students would document, on client records, all aspects of the nursing process in which they participated. At the beginning of each semester, students draft their notes for faculty review before recording on the chart, but later they document directly onto the record. Nurse practitioner staff discuss what aspects of the care provided to the client they will document, such as results of physical assessment, medical diagnoses, selected client education, or referrals. When the student finishes recording, the faculty cosigns the record, and it is placed on the nurse practitioner's desk for additional notes.

Learning Strategies

Service-learning includes a strong reflective component where students use higher-order thinking skills to make sense of and extend the formal learning for the service experience. The reflective component of the Community Health Nursing Practicum is accomplished through three learning strategies: (1) weekly informal clinical logs, (2) a formal clinic critique paper, and (3) weekly clinical seminars. The informal clinical logs assignments require the student to identify two or three of the course outcomes that they believe they addressed or accomplished during clinical work that week. The student describes in narrative form the activities that addressed the selected outcome, thus linking specific activities, such as arranging for a client to get a chest X ray at the health department, with specific learning outcomes, such as using pertinent community resources that are consistent with the client's health-care needs. In the clinical logs, students are asked to describe their reactions to their clinical experiences and to identify aspects that they think could be improved, promoting responsibility for their own learning and critical thinking regarding clinical experiences.

The formal clinic critique (see Set 2 for its guidelines) requires students to describe strengths of the clinical service, as well as barriers to delivery of services for staff and barriers to receipt of services for clients. Students conclude their paper with concrete and practical recommendations for improving clinical services. This paper requires students to use critical-thinking skills to evaluate services and creative decision making in order to identify practical approaches for improving existing services. At times, the recommendations in these papers have provided useful suggestions that have been implemented by faculty and staff at the JCDTC.

The weekly seminars associated with this Community Health Nursing Practicum provide the third opportunity for reflective learning. As in any traditional postclinical conference, students share their individual experiences in the clinic and then explore the relationship between those experiences and theoretical concepts and practices of community health. Alternate approaches to difficult situations, realities of the current health-care structure, and the larger social realities that impact homeless clients are discussed.

However, unlike traditional postconferences, students also spend significant time reflecting on their personal strengths and resources and relating them to the strengths and needs of homeless clients for whom they have provided care. (See Set 2 for excerpts.) Students explore perceived differences and similarities between themselves and the clients in order to learn how to work as partners with clients in the clinic. Students express surprise at the extent of the problem of homelessness within their own community, are often distressed and upset by the lack of resources available to meet the needs of this population, and consistently identify a breaking down of stereotypes about homeless individuals as one of their greatest insights during this course. One student recently summed up her experience by stating it gave her "a totally different perspective on people and their life experiences." Options for social activism through local government and organizations are often explored, as well as implications of current policy making at a national level. It is not uncommon at the end of the course for students to offer to return to the clinic in an elective role, or to state that they will seek opportunities to serve this population when they settle into their new graduate nursing positions.

Conclusion

Policies regarding our nation's health care are at the forefront of today's social and economic concerns. The movement of health care out of hospitals, coupled with shifting financial support for human services to state and local governments, makes service-learning a necessity rather than a luxury. Because states and local governments are often unable to fully support needed community services, there will be an ongoing and increasing need for volunteers and community service. At the same time, nursing education faces a mandate to move baccalaureate education into the community. Service-learning methods that educate about community needs and concerns, as well as about provision of care within communities, will go far toward future solutions to these issues.

The quality of campus and community partnerships will soar as a result of a service-learning program. This is a true win-win situation for all concerned. The agency receives much-needed support, the student receives a hands-on learning experience, and the college of nursing tests its curriculum through student applications in real-world situations. Beyond these obvious benefits, a multidimensional group of partnerships emerges: Faculty and health-care agencies collaborate on curricular changes; students and faculty partner in a reflective learning process; the agencies and the students partner to develop citizen-leaders; Student Affairs and Academic Affairs partner to support an experiential learning program; the client and the student engage in a mutual lesson in diversity; the student partners with another student to compare service experiences and to share ideas for social change.

The collaboration of multiple departments and divisions on campus results not only in a high-quality service-learning program but also in a more holistic approach to the learning process. Students participating in service-learning programs have the benefit of an integrated learning process, resulting in higher involvement in the process.

References

Kendall, J.C., and Associates. (1990). *Combining Service and Learning: A Resource Book for Community and Public Service.* Vol. 1. Raleigh, NC: National Society for Internships and Experiential Education.

Macnee, C.L., J.C. Hemphill, and J. Letran. (1996). "Evaluation of Outcomes of Screening Clinics for Homeless and Indigent." *Journal of Community Health Nursing* 13(3): 181-191.

A Case Study in Service-Learning Using a Collaborative Community-Based Caring Model

by Evelyn C. Atchison and Patricia A. Tumminia

As the paradigm shift in health-care delivery changes from the acute-care setting to more cost-effective care alternatives, the emphasis on community-based services and health promotion and disease prevention becomes paramount. In response to these challenges, the Division of Health Technologies at Northern Virginia Community College (NVCC), where nursing is one of eight programs within the division, received grant funding from the Corporation for National Service (Learn and Serve America). This funding supports the implementation of a community-based clinical practice, the Mobile Nurse Managed Health Center (MNMHC).

The purpose of the MNMHC is to develop a demonstration model of community-based clinical practice incorporating service-learning as a part of nursing curricula at the associate's degree level. As an outreach effort focusing on community, cultural, physical, and social needs, NVCC nursing and allied health students provide primary health-care services to special populations in the Northern Virginia area. Nursing students from local universities also utilize the MNMHC as a clinical practice site.

The program design of the MNMHC is based upon the need to effect change in educating health-care practitioners so that they will develop an appreciation for the connection between their community service activities and the underlying issues of the social problems being addressed. It is our goal for students to change their focus toward the needs of others in the community so that they gain a sense of civic and social awareness.

A major motivation toward incorporating service-learning at the associate's degree level is found in the National League for Nursing's A Vision for Nursing Education (1993). This document identifies the emerging community-based structures that will challenge academic programs to bring together the various constituencies concerned with the education of new health-care professionals, including students from associate's degree nursing (ADN) programs.

ADN faculty and students at NVCC have taken the lead in the growing movement toward community-based care via the MNMHC. The refocusing of ADN education toward community settings requires a major readjustment of nursing curricula. In order to illustrate the breadth of the change, Figure 1 shows the differences between the former nursing curriculum and

Figure 1

Difference Between Nursing Curriculum and Nursing Service-Learning Curriculum

Former Nursing Curriculum	Current Nursing Service-Learning Curriculum
1. Faculty-designed clinical practica	1. Student-designed clinical practica
2. Community service activities are voluntary, with no follow-up.	2. Community service activities are a structured part of the Reflective Educational Curriculum framework.
3. A small number of clinical rotations include community-based service, but are only observational.	3. Formalized weekly clinical rotations occur as part of the MNMHC, which are interactive, hands-on community services.
4. Clinical practica are hospital controlled.	4. Clinical practica are client/population controlled.
5. Focus is on leadership and management in the hospital setting.	5. Focus is on identification of unmet needs in the community and ways as change agents to positively influence meeting those needs.
6. Students focus on costs and quality.	6. Students focus on accessing quality care for clients.
7. Nursing practice based on Modified Primary Functional Care delivery model.	7. Nursing practice based on Differentiated Practice - Interdisciplinary Team delivery model.
8. Students focus on individual clients and their community, cultural, and social needs, and how they affect the patient.	8. Students focus on the client's community, cultural, and social needs, and relate unmet needs as causative agents to the disease processes.
9. Students focus on the acute or episodic aspects of illness.	9. Students focus on assessment and health promotion and disease prevention.

the present nursing service-learning curriculum. This comparison can be used as a model for change toward implementation of community-based care in other ADN programs.

Service-Learning

Blending service-learning with nursing education is natural, since they share common conceptual characteristics. Nursing education provides opportunities for learning that are service oriented; the expected outcome of these service activities is that students will be able to safely apply nursing theory to practice. However, the question frequently asked of nurse educators is whether the emphasis is placed on learning or service. Often, nursing educators feel that if there is a service component to the learning experience, then it can be called service-learning.

Several disciplines characterize approaches such as volunteer and community service projects, internship programs, and field studies as service-learning. The test is to determine how professional/occupational programs with service components meet the actual intent of service-learning.

Consistent with the guiding definition for this monograph (see p. 9), Robert Sigmon (1979) defines service-learning as an experiential learning approach that is premised on "reciprocal learning." Under this definition, service-learning may not apply to most nursing education programs. Timothy Stanton (1987) asked, "How do we distinguish service-learning from . . . other forms of experiential education?" (2).

Sigmon's typology of service-learning (1994) offers the best opportunity to distinguish among different types of service-learning approaches and/or programs (Figure 2). The typology helps to define the primary beneficiary and where the emphasis in the approach is placed. In most approaches, either service or learning has more weight, with more emphasis placed on one or the other. The actual intent of service-learning is that service and learning are equal in weight *and* emphasis. According to Furco (1996), "Service-learning programs must have some academic context [that] must be designed to ensure that both service enhances the learning, and learning enhances the service" (5). Therefore, nursing educators need to develop both student and client outcomes to ensure that equal weight and emphases are placed on both service and learning.

For example, in the service-learning demonstration project at Northern Virginia Community College, the expected student outcomes are that the student will develop an appreciation for community service, explore community-based careers, provide competent health-care services to diverse populations, and strengthen collaborative relationships. The expected outcomes for the recipients of the service provided are that the clients will

Figure 2

A Service and Learning Typology

service-LEARNING	Learning goals primary, service outcomes secondary
SERVICE-learning	Service outcomes primary, learning goals secondary
service-learning	Service and learning goals completely separate
SERVICE-LEARNING	Service and learning goals of equal weight, and each enhances the other for all participants

Source: Sigmon 1994

develop self-care skills and attitudes, utilize appropriate community resources to meet health-care needs, and assume primary responsibility for health-care decisions. These outcomes meet the test for the actual intent of service-learning, since the program is designed to benefit both the student who provides the service and the community recipients for whom the service is provided (Furco 1996).

Guiding Framework

Three conceptual areas were integrated into the framework for this service-learning program that addressed the unique features of the participating groups. The three conceptual areas are (1) differentiated practice in nursing, (2) the caring model, and (3) reflective framework.

Differentiated Practice in Nursing

The blending of academic study and community service provides for many structured service-learning experiences. One of our student outcomes is to strengthen collaborative relationships; therefore, we chose to approach our demonstration project through a differentiated practice model to accomplish this objective.

Differentiated nursing practice can be defined as "the practice of structuring nursing roles on the basis of education, experience, and competence" (Boston 1990). According to the report of the AACN-AONE Task Force (1995), three strategies are necessary to implement differentiated practice: (1) maximum utilization of each individual's talents; (2) application of principles of differentiation and mutually valued practice; and (3) resocialization of nurses to value and understand the "whole" of nursing's work.

Collaborative relationships among nurses and other health-care providers must be based on mutual valuing, in that each person's competence and expertise is recognized and respected. The real test in implementing the differentiated practice model is matching the health-care provider's different and unique capabilities with the client's different and unique health-care needs. The goal is to define the role of each provider so that each provider will contribute in some way to the client's care (AACN-AONE 1995).

The service-learning demonstration project at Northern Virginia Community College utilizes the Mobile Nurse Managed Health Center as a means for students to provide accessible health-care services within the community. A variation of the differentiated practice model is used where there is horizontal differentiation between nursing and allied health students at the associate's degree level and a vertical differentiation among three levels of nursing students: nurse practitioner students at the master's degree level, baccalaureate nursing students, and associate's degree nursing students. A horizontal differentiation is one in which students from a variety of health-related disciplines contribute to the client's care needs at a comparable skill level. A vertical differentiation among three levels of nursing students is one in which each skill level is more complex than the previous and requires more educational preparation.

The MNMHC is managed by a full-time family nurse practitioner (FNP) and staffed by three part-time nurse practitioners, one physician, a physician's assistant, and a van coordinator. Nursing faculty are also part of the interdisciplinary team carrying responsibility for the overall instruction and supervision of students. The role of each health-care provider is developed by the team through the formation of a job description. Roles of students are defined according to the current literature on differentiation of roles and applied to student competencies and objectives for learning. Using roles related to communication, examples of each role would be as follows:

> Associate's degree nursing (ADN) students would use basic communication skills with clients (interview the client) and utilize other team members as resources for assistance and support; baccalaureate nursing (BSN) students would use complex communication skills (teach the client) and collaborate with health team members regarding the client's care; master's degree (MSN) students would integrate and coordinate the client's care given by the ADN and BSN students as well as provide for the continuity of care for each client. (AACN-AONE 1995: 31)

The Caring Model

Defining role differences among health-care providers and valuing each person on the team are essential components to strengthening collaborative relationships. The one constant personal quality that must be shared by the entire interdisciplinary team and projected to the client is caring. Valuing and respecting each person is a form of caring. Students learn best about caring when they are placed in a caring environment. Caring qualities and/or attitudes among members of the interdisciplinary team (including faculty members) help students transfer human caring from self and the team to the client (Watson 1988). People need each other in a caring way; however, this need is often overlooked in the work setting. Caring relationships among health-care team members are essential to getting the work done in an efficient, orderly manner. Team members serve as role models for students when caring for clients in a "caring" way.

Reflective Framework

A major component of this experience is the emphasis placed on the students' social responsibility and commitment to community-based service. The structured service-learning experiences include exposure to specific populations. Students participating in service-learning activities not only provide direct community service but also learn about the context in which the service is provided. They come to understand the connection between service and their academic coursework. Students are given the opportunity to assess, teach, monitor, interview, make referrals, and write client action plans based on the uniqueness of the client. Students are assigned special responsibilities related to client care and health problems that include assessment of the problem, analysis of the problem, developing goals and objectives to respond to the problem, responding to the problem, and, finally, evaluating the results from the actions taken.

Faculty supervise all aspects of the students' service-learning experience. They hold pre- and postconferences daily to facilitate students' reflection on the experiences as a whole and on individual client problems. These reflections are shared among all students in the group, which enables them to collectively use critical-thinking skills to resolve immediate threats to an individual's or the community's health and welfare. Students develop written assignments on the service experience according to structured guidelines that include reflective and caring processes.

Critical reflective thinking by nursing students is a key factor in the service-learning project, but it is a learned skill. According to Silcox (1993), reflection "engages the individual in a cycle of thought and action based on experience, introspection, shared and examined analysis, and finally synthesis" (46). In order to develop the reflective/caring process, the student can be prepared to develop reflective/caring competencies prior to his or her community service by the case study approach. This is the first step in the community service-learning project.

Use of Case Studies in Service-Learning

At the beginning of the community experience, a case study is presented to the students in two parts. A series of progressive questions for reflection are posed for further inquiry of the client's caring needs. A set of videos on community-based care is assigned prior to the case study to enhance the students' sensitivity and awareness for reflection. Students begin to work with the case study questions in small groups in order to encourage collaboration among the group members. Students may consult textbooks or complete a library search to arrive at the answers. Discussion of the case study is facilitated by the faculty. From the case study approach, the students learn how to reflect and develop the ability to analyze client and community data. The case study allows the student to learn how to ask questions and how to create a client action plan (Figure 3), extending it to a community action plan

(Figure 4). Creativity is enhanced by having the students develop a flow chart of services for their client (Figure 5). The clients' language barriers are addressed via the students' development of a series of questions in each particular language in order to facilitate assessment of client and community needs.

As the students immerse themselves in the actual service-learning experience, they are expected to develop a portfolio assessment of their service-learning experience. The portfolio includes development of a case study of their client coupled with community action plans and questions that they formulated from the reflection/caring process. Collaboration with fellow students, staff, and faculty, and focus groups create information to share regarding service-learning through community-based care. This is a continuous process throughout the experience.

The Case Study (Part 1)

Maria Z. is a 23-year-old Hispanic woman with a strong Catholic upbringing. She is currently a college student who works part-time as a maid and uses public transportation. She was born in Merida, Mexico, on the Yucatan peninsula. Her family emigrated to the United States when she was 12 years old. The primary language spoken in her home is Spanish; however, Maria speaks English fairly well. Her family uses folk doctors, or *curanderos,* for their health problems. Maria has come to the Mobile Nurse Managed Health Center reluctantly and verbalizes her need to see a healthcare provider to examine a small sore on her labia that will not go away with the folk medicine that she has been using. She states that she is afraid that the sore may be from sexual activity and that she may have AIDS. She reveals that she and her fiancé of three years have been sexually active and have not used any protection. She also states that she has a history of asthma and chronic sinusitis and had spent four days in the hospital for pneumonia when she was 18 years old. She is currently taking Ritalin and Paxil.

Maria resides in a low-income apartment complex known as Stone Point. The population is multicultural, including Hispanic, Asian, African-American, and Caucasian families. Many residents are non–English speaking and include newly immigrated families who qualify for county-supported assistance programs. Programs available include transportation to medical clinics, free nutrition-education programs, free alcohol and drug abuse prevention programs, Meals on Wheels for homebound residents, and free counseling for filing medical assistance forms.

An interdisciplinary team at the MNMHC under the direction of the family nurse practitioner was assigned to work with Maria. The ADN student nurse interviewed Maria and took her history and vital signs. The nurse practitioner student performed the physical assessment and evaluated

Figure 3

Client Action Plan

Client Initials __MZ__ Age __23__ General Statement of Present Health Status __"Sore on labia"; fear AIDS; weight loss__
Community Site __Stone Point, Fairview County__
Previous Health History __Asthma since 17 years old, chronic sinusitis, 1992, anemia since 12 years old__
Current Medications: __Paxil, Ritalin__

Client Assessment and Unmet Needs List	Nursing Actions	Client Short- and Long-Term Goals	Follow-up/Resource Needs
Level of stress r/t, concern about AIDS	Decrease patient's level of stress through communication	To decrease her anxiety by doing the blood work she requested and referring her to a clinic	Referred to Planned Parenthood for further support for follow-up related to STD/HIV prevention
Wants HIV test and pelvis exam for unknown sore on labia	Draw blood for HIV ab and HBS-Ag testing	To have her return to the clinic on 2-28-96 to follow up on her lab results and, if negative, to return in 3 months for retest	Follow-up at clinic for results of her blood work. Return for testing in 3 months if 1st test negative.
Concerned of possibility of STDs	Teach to use condoms to decrease the possibility of STD transmission		Follow-up at clinic for results
Weight loss	Evaluate diet for nutrition assessment		
History of asthma and sinusitis	Review preventive measures used by client to prevent asthma and sinusitis		
Uses Paxil and Ritalin	Evaluate use of Paxil and Ritalin		

Figure 4

Service-Learning
Community-Based Care Plan Guidelines

Client Initials __MZ__   Age __23__

Long-Term Client Desired Outcomes

1. to use barrier methods for sexual relations
2. to follow up at clinic for results of lab work, with return for retesting in 3 months

Date	
Assessment	Content from 13-block assessment that validates and identifies causative and contributing factors of client unmet needs

Unmet Needs	1. Client micro unmet needs related to your client must be stated in approved terminology, prioritized in order of importance, and show etiology.
	2. Community macro
	  a. Existing community resources
	  b. Access issues
	  c. Health service delivery needs

Desired Outcome	Written in measurable terms toward goal attainment. Give target dates for attainment.
Client Action Plan	1. Nursing actions to help the client achieve the desired outcomes. Must be specific and individualized for your client. 2. Address the ways to effect change in relation to the causative or contributing factors of the client's unmet needs.
Rationale	Underlying reason for each nursing action; requires a reference from professional literature.
Evaluation	1. Show progress toward the desired outcomes. Use specific client data to document progress toward the desired outcome. 2. Make an evaluative statement based on follow-up visits made by P.H.N. or yourself. 3. Evaluate your service-learning experience in both the immediate and long-term perspective.

Figure 5

Flow of Services

Client: Maria

Initial Interview and History	Nursing Assessment
Associate's Degree Student	Nurse Practitioner and Nurse Practitioner Student

Respiratory Assessment	Diagnostic Testing
Respiratory Therapy Student	Medical Lab Student and Nurse Practitioner

Education	Nutrition	Stress Management	Medication Evaluation	Life-Style
BSN and ADN Nursing Student	BSN and ADN Student	BSN and ADN Student	Nurse Practitioner	ADN and BSN Nursing Student

Economic Resources	Access to Transportation
ADN and BSN and Public Health Dept.	ADN and BSN and Public Health Dept.

Recording and Reporting
Health Information Technology Student

Follow-up Planning
Interdisciplinary Team

Maria's past history and current medications. The FNP examined the sore on Maria's labia and asked for blood to be drawn. The BSN student developed a teaching plan and included appropriate referrals after speaking with the FNP. The medical lab student drew blood and sent the specimen to the laboratory, the respiratory therapy student performed an in-depth assessment of Maria's respiratory status regarding her asthma history, and the health information technology student recorded all the results from the history, assessments, and blood reports. The ADN and BSN students were asked to provide the follow-up to Maria's progress.

Questions that need to be considered by the interdisciplinary team/focus groups are:

1. What are some of the issues that Maria presents to you at this time?

2. What are some of the observations/issues that need to be considered before information is gathered regarding her health history and health assessment findings?

3. How does her cultural background impact on her health problem?

4. How does the Stone Point housing complex impact on her health?

5. What are some of the possible solutions to Maria's problems? What steps are needed to implement the solutions?

6. What services are available through Fairview County that would assist Maria with her medical and/or family problems?

7. What are some guidelines that may be needed to be effective in providing appropriate services for Maria?

8. How will the interdisciplinary team ensure continuity of care for Maria?

9. Are the roles appropriate for each team member? How could the team collaborate to provide the best care for Maria?

The Case Study Continues (Part 2)

As the nurse practitioner student assists the FNP with the assessment of the sore on her labia, Maria states that her fiancé has admitted to having unprotected sex with other women. Maria's mother says that she should not judge him, as he will be her husband in six months. As the assessment continues, the student and the FNP observe bruising on Maria's back and shoulders. Maria tearfully tells them that her fiancé thinks that she has been disobedient toward him and deserves to be punished. Her mother agrees with him. Maria tells them that, to calm down, she has been taking Paxil, given to her by her fiancé, and Ritalin, given to her by her girlfriends, so that she could go to work and attend her classes, but she continues to feel tired. She has lost a lot of weight, and her mother is worried that her wedding dress will not fit her and has started her on a tonic.

1. What are the issues that are now emerging? How will the caring con-

cepts enter into the delivery of care for Maria?

2. What is the role of women in the Hispanic culture? Can you relate to this role, or do you find it distressing? Are there any similarities to your lifestyle?

3. What is the influence of folk medicine with the Hispanic culture? How can the FNP deal with Maria's use of folk medicine? How do we show respect for others' use of folk medicine?

4. What is the influence of Maria's mother? What considerations would the care givers need to make? How can we demonstrate caring for Maria and for her mother?

5. How can care givers develop a caring attitude toward clients such as Maria?

6. What services can the team provide for Maria in order to indicate that there is sensitivity toward her role in the Hispanic society? What caring approach will be best for Maria as she deals with the fear of having AIDS?

7. What is the caring role relationship that needs to be established to ensure successful follow-up care for Maria?

Summary

Case studies are effective teaching tools that can be used to demonstrate the actual intent of service-learning. They provide students an opportunity to prepare for the community experience by exposing them to real or potential community needs. Case studies simulate client health problems that can provide an avenue for reflection from which students develop client action plans. Through the client action plans, students learn to incorporate client outcomes of care. Critical reflection of the individual client's health-care problem when placed in the context of the broader community helps students view the breadth of the health needs of the community.

Students can serve as change agents when they focus on the health-care needs of the total population and as a group create community action plans based on the aggregate of client action plans. Students can make a difference in the clients' ability to seek appropriate health care and help them gain the knowledge necessary to become empowered to make appropriate decisions about their own care needs.

A survey of ADN students who participated in community-based care at the MNMHC demonstrates that student outcomes were realized. Students responded overwhelmingly positively to the experience with regard to feeling comfortable and confident in providing primary and preventive care to clients in a community-based setting, they appreciated the difficulty clients have in finding affordable health-care services, they appreciated the effects of culture on health care, they identified role differences of various health-care providers and the need for positive working relationships, they demonstrated an interest in the community setting as a potential career choice, they identified a need for sensitivity toward clients and their lack of knowledge, and, finally, they believed that they were able to effect change to some degree through their interventions.

References

AACN-AONE Task Force. (1995). *A Model for Differentiated Nursing Practice.* Washington, DC: American Association of Colleges of Nursing.

Boston, C. (1990). "Differentiated Practice: An Introduction." In *Current Issues and Perspectives on Differentiated Practice,* edited by C. Boston, 1-3. Chicago, IL: American Organization of Nurse Executives.

Furco, A. (1996). "Service-Learning: A Balanced Approach to Experiential Education." In *Expanding Boundaries: Serving and Learning,* 2-5. Washington, DC: Corporation for National Service.

National League for Nursing. (1993). *A Vision for Nursing Education.* New York, NY: National League for Nursing.

Sigmon, R.L. (Spring 1979). "Service-Learning: Three Principles." *Synergist, National Center for Service Learning ACTION* 8(1): 9-11.

————. (1994). "Serving to Learn, Learning to Serve." In *Linking Service With Learning.* Washington, DC: Council of Independent Colleges.

Silcox, H.C. (1993). *A How-to Guide to Reflection: Adding Cognitive Learning to Community Service Programs.* Philadelphia, PA: Brighton Press.

Stanton, T. (January/February 1987). "Service Learning: Groping Toward a Definition." *Experiential Education* 12(1): 2-4.

Watson, J. (1988). "A Case Study: Curriculum in Transition." In *Curriculum Revolution: Mandate for Change,* edited by E. O. Bevis. New York, NY: National League for Nursing Press.

Community Empowerment Through Service-Learning

by Leanne C. Busby, Cathy Taylor, and Linda Norman

One strategy for preventing the reality shock that advanced-practice nursing students often experience following graduation is to expose them to situations that require critical thinking while developing sound problem-solving skills. Experiential service-learning activities that meet needs identified by communities through academic assignments can assist in this process. This paper will describe a community empowerment project that has afforded experiential service-learning activities within the Vanderbilt University School of Nursing (VUSN) curriculum. The link between service-learning activities and the development of theory-based practitioners who readily use critical-thinking skills will be examined.

The Vine Hill Community Empowerment Project

As VUSN faculty developed practice sites, a medically underserved, impoverished community 15 minutes from the university campus was brought to our attention. The Vine Hill public housing complex is home to approximately 950 individuals, about one-half of whom are children and adolescents. Ninety-three (93) percent of the families are headed by a single female. Thirty-four (34) percent of residents are between 0 and 12 years old, 13 percent are between 13 and 20, 37 percent are between 21 and 61, and 16 percent are over 62 years of age. Community residents are predominantly Caucasian. Average annual per capita income is $4,860. Average monthly rent is $99.16, with an unemployment rate above the national average.

A community-needs assessment indicated that a nurse practitioner–managed primary-care clinic would meet multiple needs: Vine Hill residents would gain better access to primary health care and other nursing resources; VUSN students would gain critical-thinking skills and a clearer understanding of theory-based practice through participation in service-learning activities with disadvantaged, medically underserved individuals and families; and VUSN faculty would gain access to a practice site where objectives of the graduate program would be met.

With initial funding from the W.K. Kellogg Foundation, the Vine Hill Community Clinic (VHCC) opened in January 1991. This nurse practitioner–managed clinic provides comprehensive primary and psychiatric–mental health care to Vine Hill residents as well as other disadvantaged populations throughout Nashville. In addition, the VHCC has served as a pivotal point for the community empowerment outreach efforts of VUSN students and faculty, which have resulted in multiple service-learning opportunities. Further opportunities for service-learning activities resulted when the Fall Hamilton School-Based Nursing Center (FHSBNC) opened as a satellite of the VHCC in July 1995.

Faculty at VUSN subscribe to the belief that community empowerment efforts supported by service-learning activities can occur only after communities define their problems and that problem solving should revolve around solutions proposed by the community (Grace 1990). Thus, the Vine Hill project was designed to deliver more than traditional health-care services. VUSN student and faculty involvement with numerous community, civic, and church groups in planning and implementing activities not only impacts the health of Vine Hill residents but also facilitates VUSN's access to a community with special needs and to individuals and families who share those needs. As a result, students have numerous opportunities to apply theory to practice through service-learning activities and develop critical-thinking skills while providing numerous services to this impoverished community.

Theory-to-Practice Linkage

Service-learning activities provide a rich opportunity to demonstrate a linkage between theory and practice and a method for the development of critical thinkers who consider social responsibilities as an integral part of their nursing practice (Tanner 1996). While in the classroom, students learn that theory predicts, describes, and/or explains some phenomena. When students enter the practice arena, the theoretical knowledge they possess helps them shape questions and systematically examine a series of events (Benner 1984). Thus, as Brookfield (1987) suggests, critical-thinking skills emerge as students identify and challenge assumptions, challenge the importance of context, and imagine and explore alternatives, while considering their own perspectives as well as perspectives of others. These traits, when developed, result in thoughtful analysis of identified needs with acknowledgment of individual perceptions along with logical, goal-directed, problem-solving approaches (Watson and Glaser 1980). The theory-to-practice linkage, then, is evident in at least three ways: (1) Theory provides a frame of reference for practice; (2) theory provides a method whereby practical events can be analyzed; and (3) theory provides the knowledge upon which practical, logical decisions are made (Hoy and Miskel 1978).

Student Involvement

Since the project began, more than 395 graduate nursing, medical, and social work students have experienced a four- to 12-week clinical rotation in the Vine Hill community. Originally, family nurse practitioner (FNP) graduate students were involved with Vine Hill residents through clinical rotations at the VHCC. As community empowerment efforts expanded, it quickly became obvious that there was much more for students to experience than *just* the delivery of traditional primary health care. Thus, the idea of introducing students to the concept of critical thinking and strengthening their theory-based practice experience through service-learning activities with Vine Hill residents emerged.

In order for service-learning activities to impact community empowerment, faculty and students were committed to the assumption that the community had to define the problem and propose solutions. This concept, which is not always practiced by health-care professionals, was best accomplished by first bringing together those who share a common problem. As proposed by Grace (1990), our students served as a catalytic force entering the community and asking key questions. Then community residents were able to clarify specific issues and outline steps toward solving problems.

We also acknowledged that to increase problem-solving capacity of the community, small successes must build on one another to achieve a broad impact. As problems are mastered and successes and competence are achieved, community members are encouraged to move on to solving new problems. We had to also remember that inability to achieve success did not always signal defeat (Grace 1990). As with successful programs, critical evaluation of programmatic failures has resulted in rich student learning experiences.

For students, theoretical knowledge needs to be further enhanced through experiential learning, which has been described by Burnard (1987) as knowledge that is gained through direct personal interactions with people, subjects, or things. We have seen, as suggested by Rogers (1969), that quality personal involvement, self-initiation, and meaningfulness to the learner are all elements of experiential learning that are essential in the development of theory-based practice. This community empowerment project has resulted in a clear portrait of the theory-to-practice linkage as described below.

Community Interagency Collaboration

Community interagency collaboration has been noted to facilitate pooling of resources and mutual goal achievement (Alter and Hage 1993; Polivka 1995). *Healthy Communities 2000: Model Standards* (American Public Health Association 1991) describes the fundamental importance of shared, public- and private-sector partnerships among major community groups and organizations in achieving disease-prevention goals for the nation. Though time- and labor-intensive to initiate and maintain, this approach involves mobilization of community leaders, identification of agencies serving similar populations (e.g., the YMCA), and recruitment of nontraditional sources of manpower and funding (e.g., local businesses) for pursuit of agreed-upon goals.

An example of this occurred when faculty and students mentored Vine Hill residents as they established the Vine Hill Volunteers (VHVs). The goal of this community group, organized in 1991, is "a better life for our kids." Designating job training and skill development of parents and care givers as the preferred route to this end, the group also focuses on development and implementation of children's programs. As students provided and facilitated training in leadership, life skills, and job training and placement, many reported a preconceived notion that "welfare recipients were lazy and lacked motivation." Having never worked with minimally skilled, moderately educated adults, students described how their perceptions about "welfare moms" were challenged. Those students progressing as critical, reflective thinkers describe how their perceptions have changed over time. Further, they consistently demonstrate a unique ability to consider opposing viewpoints (Bandman and Bandman 1995) as they reflect on their own preconceived perceptions and personal biases while assisting the community in problem solving. As families in the community realize personal and community goals for success, the students' efforts are recognized, leading to even more reflective thinking. We believe this develops a graduate who exercises outstanding clinical judgment, as suggested by Facione, Facione, and Sanchez (1994).

VUSN faculty and students also worked with the VHVs in forming the Vine Hill Children's Coalition. The purpose of this organization, as determined by community residents, is to increase the recognition of community needs by various resource agencies and groups throughout the greater Nashville area, particularly the needs of community children. Meetings, facilitated by VUSN faculty and students, occur every other month. Efforts of the coalition have resulted in ongoing summer and after-school enrichment programs sponsored by the YMCA, Girl Scouts, area churches, and other businesses. As problems arise and students assist community residents to analyze the problem and reach logical solutions, Brookfield's (1987) assumption that the development of critical-thinking skills is an ongoing process and not just an outcome of the educational experience is supported.

In 1995, VUSN faculty and students collaborated with the metropolitan Nashville juvenile court system to develop a juvenile delinquency program to target Vine Hill children at risk. As a result of this program, VUSN students have implemented "Kelso's Choice," a commercially available conflict-management curriculum, to address behavior problems at Fall Hamilton Elementary School. After the first pilot of "Kelso's Choice," teachers reported dramatic decreases in fighting and violent behavior among participants. This program has been expanded to include other classrooms and continues to have successful outcomes.

Ongoing interagency community collaboration is one crucial element in the development of students with critical-thinking skills. Successful pooling of resources with mutual goal achievement for all participants and nontraditional, positive networking and collaboration leads students to reflect on this lived experience in order to clarify its meaning (Boyd and Fales 1983). As the experience is explored, an increased sensitivity to the environment emerges, and increased self-awareness often occurs along with a change in perception (Baker 1996).

Other Service-Learning Activities

In addition to formal opportunities to participate in interagency collaborative efforts to positively impact health outcomes in the Vine Hill community, many other service-learning experiences have occurred. Students are encouraged and recruited to participate in the project through faculty presentations in various course meetings, through interviews with faculty and the clinical placement coordinator, and through word of mouth from previous students. Oftentimes, the students choosing to participate in this project are reflective, thoughtful people who enjoy the challenge of new experiences.

Community health nursing students work with faculty, Vine Hill families, and area agencies to update the baseline community assessment each semester and to design and implement health-promotion/disease-prevention projects based on outcomes of the assessment. Using Burnard's (1987) proposed four-stage experiential learning model of nursing education, students initially receive theoretical and practical information (Stage 1) regarding "community as client" concepts, community assessment, and data-collection and interviewing techniques. This includes a "windshield survey" of the community, a "ride-along" experience with neighborhood police, and an introduction to vital statistics and census data retrieval as well as introductions to community leaders and service agency representatives. Community assessment tools are used to guide data collection, and student experiences are shared during small-group clinical seminars. Early evidence of developing critical-, reflective-thinking skills is seen as students identify strengths and problem areas, and begin to reflect on unique and shared experiences resulting from the assignment (Stage 2).

Data collection is completed and facilitated with regular seminars involving faculty and students for continued reflection and discussion regarding processes and outcomes of each level of activity (Stage 3). Learning is further enhanced with field trips to the state legislature to hear testimony regarding policy development impacting the Vine Hill population. As suggested by Boyd and Fales (1983), students share that this experiential learning activity has impacted their view of themselves and the world. Oftentimes, they express surprise at their own growth, which they had not recognized while so intimately involved in interactions with communities and families.

Student projects such as fire and in-home safety, dental hygiene, management of lice and cockroach infestations, gun and pedestrian safety, and preschool developmental screening and intervention have been developed and implemented based on completed assessment and analysis of data. Low-literacy, educational materials on such topics as insect bites, skin rashes, constipation and diarrhea, fever, earaches, and "bumps to the head" have been developed by students and are disseminated through the FHSBNC newsletter. Once again, students consistently report a personal changing worldview as they reflect on these experiential service-learning activities.

Students also make home visits and complete a family assessment using the Calgary Family Assessment Model described by Wright and Leahy (1994). Prior to this activity, students are introduced to the concepts of poverty and health, trust building, working with multiproblem families, and identification of family strengths.

At the conclusion of these activities, students and faculty evaluate the learning experience and plan future application to practice (Stage 4). Students not only outline strengths and weaknesses of the experience and describe application to their own future practice but also are charged with developing recommendations to enhance community-based outcomes and give directions for subsequent student groups. As students reflect on this experience and the link between theory and practice described earlier, they are able to demonstrate an ability to consider opposing viewpoints through an attitude of inquiry leading to logical problem solving. Many share that this approach is useful in all areas of professional nursing practice, whether the client is an individual, a family, or a community of any size.

Graduate nurse practitioner students participate in the annual Vine Hill Health Fair. They assist with numerous health-promotion/disease-prevention activities, such as cardiovascular risk screening, health and fitness screening for children, mammography for women over age 35, nutrition and fitness counseling for children and their care givers, oral hygiene and dental care education, and childhood safety education. This service-learning activity affords students opportunities to demonstrate critical-, reflective-thinking skills as they present creative ideas and programs that often become part of ongoing community activities.

For those FNP and psychiatric–mental health students who are assigned to the VHCC for clinical rotations, many other valuable lessons are learned.

These students work one on one with VUSN faculty in this preceptored learning laboratory. Unlike at some other clinical placement sites, their exposure to the needs of varying culturally diverse and impoverished individuals challenges their critical-thinking skills and facilitates their use of new and varied resources. The development of individual plans of care that consider cultural and financial differences in patients demonstrates the students' evolving critical-thinking skills.

Specific student projects can best describe how critical, reflective thinking is fostered through service-learning activities. In one situation, a group of graduate FNP students developed and implemented a patient education program related to hypertension, with education and intervention focused on blood pressure monitoring along with dietary and life-style expectations. Early on, the students were distraught when participants reported life-style habits that increased their risk for hypertension. However, as students were encouraged to develop an attitude of inquiry, they came to the realization that the real problem was lack of education rather than their original perception that patients were "ignoring" the prescribed dietary regimen. Subsequently, education/intervention focused on blood pressure monitoring along with dietary and life-style expectations, and as positive outcomes emerged, students were able to see the theory-to-practice linkage through reflective and critical thinking.

A community-based "Lullaby Club" was formed to address needs of very young mothers. The club, developed by community health nursing students with faculty mentoring, focuses on identified precursors to child abuse, strong parental beliefs in corporal punishment, and unrealistic developmental expectations of children. In this situation, students were able to apply theory to practice and work with community residents to plan for alternative approaches to child rearing. Once again, students reported reflective thinking, critical evaluation of outcomes, and logical problem-solving approaches as steps taken to plan for change.

A Blueprint for Service-Learning Activities

In order to demonstrate the theory-to-practice linkage and enhance critical, reflective thinking in students, service-learning activities must be developed and fostered. The following blueprint is suggested for faculty interested in integrating successful service-learning activities into nursing curricula:

- Step 1. Conduct a community needs assessment.
- Step 2. Delineate clear goals and expectations based on outcomes of the needs assessment as you plan service-learning activities.
- Step 3. Gain educational facility and community "buy-in." This is best accomplished through meetings in which the community confirms needs as

identified through the needs assessment.

- Step 4. Assist the community to prioritize needs and determine long- and short-range goals of all participants.
- Step 5. Consistently develop and foster relationships with community leaders and service agencies.
- Step 6. Create and foster partnerships/coalitions with agencies and community leaders.
- Step 7. Regularly measure progress toward goals.
- Step 8. Analyze failures and successes, and revise interventions.
- Step 9. Regularly update needs assessment.
- Step 10. Acknowledge and celebrate successes.

Outcomes and Lessons Learned

Student evaluations suggest an overwhelming appreciation for the opportunity to synthesize and apply theoretical knowledge through participation in service-learning activities. They express a newfound appreciation of available community services and resources and easily articulate how the comprehensive experience will impact their future roles as providers of health care and consumer advocates. The only identified disadvantage of integrating service-learning activities into the curriculum centers around time limitations. Even when families are late or fail to keep appointments, assignments must be completed during the student's assigned clinical time.

Numerous invaluable lessons have been learned as service-learning activities have been incorporated into the curriculum. Many of our own preconceived notions have been challenged, and we have often realized that what we say and teach may not always reflect what we *really* believe. When this occurs, our own critical-, reflective-thinking skills assist us to refine these notions, and our own expertise is expanded (Benner 1984).

First, we learned that service-learning activities and community-empowerment efforts have to occur within the community's time frame, in spite of the academic time frame. Second, we learned that when one has never been poor or without needed resources, it is often difficult to understand the significance of this when it occurs in others. Third, we learned that our colleagues may not always understand the time investment needed to meet goals and objectives. Fourth, we learned that meaningful outcome measurements are difficult to attain and that tools to measure whether critical, reflective thinking has occurred are either nonexistent or marginally acceptable. Fifth, we learned that competing priorities and multiple pressures only mount when service-learning activities are undertaken within the academic setting. Finally, and likely most important, we learned that community and academic needs are evolving and unless we keep the community needs as the focus of the activity, the community will not accept any services we may offer and student growth will cease.

Conclusion

The VUSN curriculum provides a logical pathway for promoting interest in community-based service-learning activities, an opportunity for students to experience the theory-to-practice linkage, and the development of critical, reflective thinking in students who will be the health-care providers of the future. Opportunities for the integration of service-learning activities in nursing curricula are abundant. Often they are labor-intensive, time-con-suming, and challenging. We believe these opportunities increase student learning, remind faculty of real-world issues, and introduce academic insti-tutions to community needs and resources. In short, as nursing education attempts to meet the expectations of a reforming health-care delivery sys-tem, service-learning activities can facilitate the development of theory-based practitioners who consistently employ reflective, critical thinking as they develop into expert practitioners.

References

Alter, C., and J. Hage. (1993). *Organizations Working Together.* Newbury Park, CA: Sage Publications.

American Public Health Association. (1991). *Healthy Communities 2000: Model Standards.* 3d ed. Washington, DC: American Public Health Association.

Baker, C.R. (1996). "Reflective Learning: A Teaching Strategy for Critical Thinking." *Journal of Nursing Education* 35(1): 19-22.

Bandman, E., and E. Bandman. (1995). *Critical Thinking in Nursing.* 2d ed. Norwalk, CT: Appleton & Lange.

Benner, P. (1984). *From Novice to Expert: Excellence and Power in Clinical Nursing Practice.* Menlo Park, CA: Addison-Wesley.

Boyd, E., and A. Fales. (1983). "Reflective Learning: Key to Learning From Experience." *Journal of Human Psychology* 23(2): 99-117.

Brookfield, S.D. (1987). *Developing Critical Thinkers.* San Francisco, CA: Jossey-Bass.

Burnard, P. (1987). "Towards an Epistemological Basis for Experiential Learning in Nurse Education." *Journal of Advanced Nursing* 12: 189-193.

Facione, N.C., P.A. Facione, and C.A. Sanchez. (1994). "Critical Thinking Disposition as a Measure of Competent Clinical Judgment: The Development of the California Critical Thinking Disposition Inventory." *Journal of Nursing Education* 33: 345-350.

Grace, H. (1990). "Building Community: A Conceptual Perspective." W.K. *Kellogg Foundation International Journal* 2(2): 7-9.

Hoy, W.K., and C.G. Miskel. (1978). *Educational Administration: Theory, Research, and Practice.* New York, NY: Random House.

Polivka, B.J. (1995). "A Conceptual Model for Community Interagency Collaboration." *Image* 27(2): 110-115.

Rogers, C.R. (1969). *Freedom to Learn.* Columbus, OH: Charles E. Merrill Publishing Co.

Tanner, C.A. (1996). "Critical Thinking Revisited: Paradoxes and Emerging Perspectives." *Journal of Nursing Education* 35(1): 3-4.

Watson, G., and E.M. Glaser. (1980). *Watson-Glaser Critical Thinking Appraisal.* Forms A and B. New York, NY: Psychological Corp.

Wright, L.M., and M. Leahey. (1994). *Nurses and Families: A Guide to Family Assessment and Intervention.* 2d ed. Philadelphia, PA: F.A. Davis Co.

Nursing Clinical Education in an Urban Public School System

by Donna Miles Curry, Kimberley X. Hickok, and Kate Cauley

Service as a Value in Nursing

The profession of nursing has long been associated with the concept of service. Service could be said to be a "helpful act" or a "contribution to the welfare of others" (*Webster's Collegiate Dictionary*, 10th ed.). The American Nurses Association in 1965 defined nursing as "a helping profession and, as such, [one that] provides services [that] contribute to the health and well-being of people" (in Taylor et al. 1993: 7).

The act of caring for or helping others is as old as civilization itself. Nursing began with family members (usually women) providing physical care and herbal treatments to their sick and/or assisting during childbirth (Taylor et al. 1997). With the advent of Christianity, the role of the nurse was more clearly defined. Women, called "deaconesses," were responsible for visiting the sick. However, not until the 17th and 18th centuries did those providing care to the ill gain recognition as "nurses."

In 1860, Florence Nightingale, considered to be the first nursing theorist and educator, developed a formalized training program for nurses (Taylor et al. 1997). Using an "apprenticeship" approach, Nightingale assigned student nurses to work with a ward sister at St. Thomas's Hospital in London (Oermann 1994). In the United States, the first professional preparation for nurses was begun in the 1870s using much the same approach Nightingale had. Student nurses as providers of care in hospitals learned "on the job." It could be said that "service rather than education" was the primary focus of most nursing education programs in the beginning (Oermann 1994: 153).

Since the 1800s, the profession of nursing has benefited from many changes in terms of both societal factors and curricular changes in educational programs. With the rapid growth of colleges and universities following World War II, hospital-based programs for educating nurses have been nearly phased out and replaced by college preparation (associate's or baccalaureate degree). Although nursing education is no longer built upon the apprenticeship model, its history of service has become an ethic of service, and service remains a central tenet in the profession and in the educational process as we move into the 21st century.

Service-learning initiatives provide a structured process that gives voice to the history, present, and future of nursing and nursing education. Additionally, within this structure the legitimization of community- and service-based learning that has so long been at the core of the tradition of nursing finds expression. In service-learning, nursing leads the way with experience and knowledge.

Service-Learning Grant as a Stimulus for the Process of Change

In 1994, when the Center for Healthy Communities, a community-academic partnership, received a grant from the Corporation for National and Community Service, the College of Nursing and Health at Wright State University, one of six health-professions schools included with the center, began its structured service-learning program. Support from the grant facilitated both a reallocation of resources in the area of community- and service-based clinical training and an expansion of clinical sites within the public school system. The goals to be met under the grant from the Corporation included (1) improving the health of the children in the community, (2) increasing community-based learning opportunities for health professions students, and (3) impacting institutions by strengthening the community-academic partnership.

The program has been strongly supported, thanks to the clear articulation of service as a value in the mission of the university. Wright State University is a metropolitan university with a commitment to providing leadership in addressing the educational, social, and cultural needs of the greater Miami valley, and promoting the economic and technological development of the region through a strong program of basic and applied research and professional service.

An important component of the grant was to move health professions students outside the walls of academic and health-care institutions and into churches, schools, homes, and community health centers, and among the people themselves, thus embodying the educational model of the "teaching community." Consistent with the profession of nursing's historical values and dedication to service, the College of Nursing and Health at Wright State University (CONH/WSU) found participation in a Learn and Serve America project in the community through the public schools very natural. With a philosophy similar to that of the program at Northeastern University (Matteson 1995), CONH/WSU has shifted the focus of clinical education away from tertiary care settings and into the community. The communities of East and West Dayton were selected to serve as the teaching community sites, partially because of their unique diversity, East Dayton being primarily a Caucasian Appalachian community and West Dayton predominantly an African-American one.

Another important component of the grant was a focus on children's health issues. Operating with the belief that a healthy child is a better learner, health professions faculty and public school officials targeted six elementary school facilities, placing special emphasis on the kindergarten population.

Funds from the grant supported the work of health professions faculty from the College of Nursing and Health, the Department of Social Work, and the Schools of Medicine and Professional Psychology from Wright State University, and the Departments of Dental Hygiene and Dietetic Technology from the Allied Health Division of Sinclair Community College. These faculty began meeting as a multiprofessional team on a weekly basis to develop service-learning opportunities for their students. These regular meetings facilitated peer support and provided a mechanism through which educational resources about service-learning and reflection could be explored and tested. Furthermore, meeting regularly as a multiprofessional team facilitated coordination of services in the six schools and provided opportunities for students to work multiprofessionally.

The first task for the multiprofessional faculty team was to explore their own experiences of service. Using structured exercises and reflection tools, the team began a faculty development program in service-learning to prepare for facilitating the experiences of their students. The faculty team developed service-learning objectives and then modified them to discipline-specific service-learning objectives. From there, courses were identified where incorporating a service-learning component would be most appropriate. In some cases, new courses were developed to facilitate student service-learning opportunities. The next step was for faculty to move into the public school setting, both to orient themselves to the schools and to orient public school personnel to the service-learning concept while identifying ways in which health professions students could be most effectively utilized in the school setting.

Overview of the Learning Experiences

The College of Nursing and Health elected to have faculty and students from its pediatric and community health courses work with the Learn and Serve America: Higher Education project. The faculty involved in the project developed and implemented nine learning objectives for the students. Implementation varied depending on the level of the student or the focus of the course. These objectives included:

- Identify differences in growth and development of school-age children.
- Observe and participate in the role and responsibilities of the school

nurse.

- Demonstrate basic competency and interpretation of health screens.
- Develop an awareness of the health needs of school-age children.
- Provide health-promotion education in collaboration with the school nurse or classroom teacher.
- Identify the impact of political, social, cultural, environmental, and economic issues on the health of school-age children.
- Collaborate with other disciplines and community resources to meet the health needs of school-age children.
- Demonstrate effective communication skills with children, families, and professionals.
- Explore ethical/legal issues related to meeting the health needs of school-age children.

The setting for these service-learning opportunities was a midsized city with a total population of 182,005 (per the 1990 census), 106,078 of whom are Caucasian, 73,748 African-American, and 2,218 "other." Like many urban cities, Dayton has lost much of its industrial base, leaving many without adequate jobs to support their families. Median family income (1990) was $24,819 and per capita income only $9,946; approximately 27 percent of families reported living below the poverty level.

The public school system has more than 2,500 children enrolled in kindergarten and a K-12 total enrollment of close to 22,000. Sixty percent of the student population is African-American. Seventy-five percent of the student population is ADC eligible. For a number of years, there has been a magnet school system in place as a means of avoiding forced busing and distributing the racial balance more evenly. Still, Dayton remains a racially and ethnically divided city.

Both junior-level pediatric and senior-level community health nursing students were involved in service-learning activities. In the first year of the program, each of more than 100 nursing students spent an average of four clinical days with school nurses and/or in kindergarten classrooms over the course of an academic quarter.

The Pediatric Experience

The Nursing of Child-Rearing Families (pediatric nursing) course is located in the curriculum at the end of the junior year. The students have three hours of lecture and nine hours of clinical work each week for the academic quarter. The pediatric students were each assigned to one school nurse in a specific building. The activities they engaged in were numerous, from assisting in routine clinic operations and health screenings to teaching health education classes (see table).

Pediatric Nursing Students' Activities
Reported by Category and Frequency of Activity

Category of Activity	Frequency of Activity
Chart Review	
Immunizations	25
Health history	33
Phone numbers	17
Screening Activity	
Eye	42
Ear	37
Dental	27
Head lice	25
Other	19
Minor Injuries	33
Asthma	17
Counseling	25
Home Visits	3
Child Abuse	19
Health Teaching	34
Neuro Checks	6
CPR	1
Major Injuries	2

Number of students reporting activities:	29

Students were asked to keep a log of their experiences and activities. They included scoliosis screening, follow-up on immunization records, interdisciplinary conferences on select student problems, and teaching informal as well as formal classes on health topics such as safety, common childhood diseases, and healthy heart activities. Some students had the opportunity to participate in large-scale screening and a formal health fair.

Though the actual clinical experiences were valuable, the real learning occurred through the extensive reflective component of the course. Students were asked to complete two different types of reflective exercises: one focusing on the school experience in general and the other focusing on critical thinking and decision making. First, in addition to recording types of experiences in their logs, students were also instructed to record on a daily basis their reflections about the experiences. Second, students were given a series of structured but open-ended questions to respond to, based on a critical-thinking model developed by Chris Tanner (1994). Questions focused on decision making in specific situations. For instance, students were asked to describe their most challenging decision, the circumstances, and what made it challenging. Several themes were seen in the types of decisions the students perceived as challenging.

Assessment issues. Students had a difficult time determining whether a child was really sick and when a child should be sent home. These decisions were particularly difficult to make when the symptoms involved allergic reactions such as wheezing or asthma, or when children complained of stomachaches, nausea, and vomiting. An unfortunately frequent concern was trying to decide when problems were due to child abuse.

Teaching issues. How to keep classroom order and discipline during a lesson was perceived as a problem. Additionally, students identified challenging decisions related to *collaboration issues.* Making appropriate referrals and identifying resources were hindered initially by lack of knowledge of the school district and community resources. Many of the students did not have experience working with organizations such as child protective services. And for several students, there were significant challenges in working with their interdisciplinary team members such as the elementary school teachers, principals, and other professionals in the system. Finally, working with parents was identified as challenging, particularly around decisions involving parental responsibilities and privacy issues.

Building on the knowledge gained through their articulation of challenges, students were then invited to develop strategies to assist them in decision making. For instance, students quickly identified monitoring symptoms as a way to determine levels of acuity in children's illnesses. In response to challenges related to teaching, students developed strategies that included using age-appropriate language and terminology kept as simple as possible. Students were given additional opportunity to reflect on their experiences when they were asked to respond to the question, What alternatives did you consider, if any, and why did you decide to do what you finally did? And finally, students were asked to identify resources they could use to assist them when trying to make difficult decisions. Interestingly, they determined it was important to gather more information and complete further assessment whenever possible. Sources of information students identified included a child's parents (to obtain a clearer picture of the family history and home life of the child), the school nurse (her professional knowledge and expertise as well as personal knowledge of the child), the child's records (background and related health history with screenings, past illnesses, allergies, etc.), other professionals, and their own experience and expertise.

The individual evaluations provided by pediatric nursing students regarding their own decisions included a number of items. Overall, students were satisfied with their responses to difficult situations (80% satisfied, 10% not satisfied, and 5% concerned). Those who indicated satisfaction with their decisions cited factors such as successful follow-up to referrals. Students' learning was remarkably evident in response to questions about what they would do differently next time. Several themes emerged:

• Use more instructional tools when providing health education, i.e., chalkboards, pictures, hands-on experiences.

• Prepare, prepare, prepare.

• Organize, organize, organize.

• Remember: Simplicity is key.

• Build in more time to develop rapport — with the children themselves, with their parents, with their teachers, with the school nurse, and with other professionals in the community.

It became clear that interpersonal skills were as valuable as physical assessment skills in providing care.

Again, several themes emerged when students were asked what they had specifically learned from this experience. The students had a clearer understanding of the responsibilities and work of the school nurse; in particular, students learned that school nurses consider all options before making decisions, most often respond to a problem with resources immediately at hand, and deal with a lot of child abuse cases. The students learned many things about children, e.g., how they frequently come to the school clinic not because of physiological needs but because of psychosocial needs, how important it is to provide a trusting environment and privacy for children when they come to talk to the school nurse, and how, for the most part, children are truthful about themselves and their problems and can be taken at their word. Finally, students learned a great deal about the "system," including the value of screening, the importance of follow-ups and referrals, and the necessity of comprehensive charting and paperwork as a constant part of the work.

The Community Health Experience

The course Community Health Nursing is at the senior level and is one in which students typically complete a comprehensive assessment of a particular neighborhood (census tract) in the community. The exercise facilitates a better understanding of the socioeconomic and demographic characteristics of a particular population, and demonstrates the impact of environmental factors on the health of individuals and their community. For the students who participated in the Learn and Serve America program, the community assessment afforded them the opportunity to learn about some of the health-related strengths and concerns of the community where the children lived and attended school.

In one of the community health sections, 14 nursing students were divided into two groups of seven and assigned to two elementary schools, one on the east side of town and one on the west side of town. Each group of seven worked in pairs and spent three clinical days involved in the project. Rather than working with individual children through the contact point of the school nurse's office, these students were assigned to a kindergarten teacher and a classroom of students with whom to work. On day one, students were in the public schools, observing and speaking with the children, their teachers, and the school nurse. Following their observations, students were asked to identify a health-related need that could be addressed through education (primary prevention). Each student pair or group selected a topic and then developed a health-promotion education presentation. On day two, students developed learning objectives and planned the health education lesson, obtaining materials and resources needed for the presentation. Students also practiced their lesson presentations. Day three brought a return to the assigned schools and an opportunity to present their health lesson in three different classrooms. Topics included hygiene/hand washing, safety, nutrition/healthy foods, and oral hygiene.

Following days one and three, students were assigned reflective exercises focused on decision making, self-analysis, and an evaluation of decisions made. Students were asked to respond to specific questions through journal-writing exercises. After the observation day and before their teaching experience, students were asked what assumptions, beliefs, or opinions of theirs were challenged by the experience. Four themes were identified and are discussed below in order of most frequently identified to least:

• Normal hygiene practices — Students were surprised to learn how poor personal hygiene was among the children and how uninformed they seemed to be about basic hygiene concerns.

• Parents' seeming lack of responsibility in caring for the children.

• Poverty/low socioeconomic status — Though they had learned the statistics prior to their school experience, students were still surprised by the extent of poverty and its significant impact on the children, particularly as manifested by their personal hygiene practices and possible signs of parental neglect.

• School behaviors — Students were surprised to learn how often children were absent from school, and they were concerned about the classroom environment in terms of general student behavior and the abilities of the children to learn and complete classroom work.

In response to a question about what health issues or concerns related to the kindergartners the students identified during the experience, students identified personal hygiene practices, absenteeism, immunizations, head lice, and oral health care as primary concerns. In an attempt to assess the impact of the service-learning experiences on cultural awareness/competence, students were asked how their knowledge and/or awareness of the cultural ethnic group had been enhanced or changed from this experience. Again, students identified the significant impact of poverty and socioeconomic status, the importance of recognizing individuals and individual differences within cultural groups, the seeming lack of attention from parents to areas such as hygiene, basic needs, and absenteeism, and some of the unique aspects of the urban Appalachian culture.

The last question they were asked after the observation day but prior to actually teaching was whether they had changed how they might approach their health education lesson/presentation as a result of the observation/experience. Student insights included:

1. Keep the presentation simple and designed for children with very short attention spans.

2. Use hands-on experience as instructional methodology using multiple teaching aids.

3. Include strategies for classroom control in the lesson plan.

After their health-education/primary-prevention teaching experiences, students were asked to reflect further on their experiences. When asked what they would do differently if they had it to do over again, students reiterated the importance of their insights from the observation day.

Student responses to a question about what they would tell a friend/peer about the experience in the public schools ranged from global observations to very specific concerns: Students were surprised to learn the extent of state and federal support being utilized by the children and their families; students reported the significance of field experiences in really bringing to life the facts learned from a textbook; and students were very impressed with the school nurses and the teachers in their fair and equal treatment of the children without regard to conditions of poverty or differences in race. Additionally, students reported their surprise at the high physical-activity level of the children, their seeming self-acceptance, and how many of them routinely struggled with head lice.

Based on their experience in the schools, community health nursing students were asked to recommend who would be best suited to provide health-education/primary-prevention lessons to the elementary school children. For the most part, they suggested that the school nurse was the most qualified but that since her time resources were limited, the next best option to develop and teach health-promotion/disease-prevention strategies to the children would be classroom teachers in collaboration with the school nurse and other health professionals.

Finally, in an attempt to improve the service-learning experiences for future community health nursing students, students were asked to make recommendations for future projects. They suggested a number of interesting topics, including lessons on infection control, developing classes in the community for parents to stress the importance of immunizations, follow-up for deficits identified during health screening, and generally getting parents more involved in the health of their children. In summary, the community health nursing students benefited from learning about the neighborhood and community surrounding the schools. Preceding the experience in the schools, the community assessment provided a context in which the nursing students could better understand and appreciate the health and psychosocial concerns of the school children. Home visits to follow up on identified health needs and to provide families with health education would strengthen the service-learning experience even more.

Conclusions

A careful evaluation of the first year of student experiences in the service-learning program through an analysis of reflective exercises and student outcomes yielded much useful information. First, there was information related to content areas that deserve special emphasis in the general curriculum. For instance, in the second year of the project, classes prior to the clinical component included greater emphasis on content areas such as teaching strategies, the impact of the culture of poverty, and how to recognize indicators of child abuse.

Second, there were broader implications for faculty and curriculum beyond the Learn and Serve America program. Faculty, especially the clinical faculty previously used to coordinating clinical experiences in acute-care facilities, need to develop more skills and greater flexibility when coordinating clinical experiences in community settings, particularly community settings where health care is not the primary function of the facility. In addition to developing greater flexibility, faculty must acknowledge their role as learners as well as teachers. They must be willing to learn about new sites and community resources and to rededicate themselves to the importance of primary care. Interestingly, but not surprisingly, the community health nursing faculty have demonstrated wider experience in this arena, and they were helpful in facilitating the transition from acute-care to primary/community-care settings for the more traditional pediatric clinical faculty.

As a result of the College of Nursing and Health's involvement in the Learn and Serve America project, the curriculum has been modified. Students now complete cultural competence assessments before and after their community-based clinical experiences. Teaching strategies for providing health education are becoming part of the curriculum. Pediatric nursing students now spend at least four days in the community with a school nurse. (This is in addition to other community-based pediatric clinical experiences.)

There have also been significant changes in the public schools as a result of the service-learning experiences. School personnel are more familiar with the abilities of the undergraduate nursing student. Teachers, generally quite careful about whom they invite to join them in the classroom, now accept the undergraduate nursing students and recognize the expertise they can bring. This has resulted in more opportunities for student placements in service- and community-based clinical settings. The school system has begun to rely on the availability of nursing students to assist with routine functions, including health screening and other health-promotion educational activities.

As nursing educators, we have an obligation to ensure that our students are better prepared for the market as service professionals. Service-learning opportunities enhance students' generalist preparation and prepare them to be better clinicians. Without a doubt, this type of clinical experience has important positive outcomes for the nursing student. It never ceases to amaze us how many students remark that they dread going to schools, how boring it will be, that it is not where the action is, that they would rather be in the hospitals. But they almost always change their tune after the experience and heartily endorse our continuing efforts to offer service- and community-based experiences for future students. Have the students learned anything? Was this a valuable experience? Was a service provided in a learning context? The answer to all of these questions is a resounding YES!

References

Matteson, P.S. (1995). *Teaching Nursing in the Neighborhoods: The Northeastern University Model*. New York, NY: Springer.

Oermann, M.H. (1994). "Professional Nursing Education in the Future: Changes and Challenges." *Journal of Obstetrical, Gynecological, and Neonatal Nursing* 23(2): 153-159.

Tanner, C. (1994). "Provocative Thoughts on Critical Thinking." *Journal of Nursing Education* 33(8): 339.

Taylor, C., C. Lillis, and C. LeMone. (1997). *Fundamentals of Nursing: The Art and Science of Nursing Care*. 3d ed. Philadelphia, PA: Lippincott.

The Community as Classroom:
Service-Learning in Tillery, North Carolina

by Nina P. Shah and Mary A. Glascoff

The purpose of this chapter is to describe the Tillery Learn&Serve Community Project (TLC) conducted by East Carolina University (ECU) under the auspices of a Learn and Serve America: Higher Education grant. The Tillery project is a multidisciplinary attempt to improve the health status of an isolated rural North Carolina community. University faculty members and students from the disciplines of nursing, medicine, occupational therapy, physical therapy, hearing and speech pathology, nutrition, environmental health, and health education, as well as members of the Tillery community, made up the team. Undergraduate, graduate, and professional students performed, and continue to perform, vital community service activities in Tillery, North Carolina, under the guidance of the ECU faculty.

Tillery's History

Tillery is a unique crossroads community of 1,500 residents located in rural Halifax County, North Carolina. During the 1930s, the Tillery area was selected to be one of 117 resettlement communities established under the Forty Acres and a Mule program as part of FDR's New Deal. Significantly, Tillery was one of only 17 resettlement communities in the country established for African-American citizens. Despite the seemingly good intentions of that program, residents of Tillery who came with the resettlement project often say, "We never saw the 40 acres, and the mule had good understanding and left." Today, 98 percent of the population of the Tillery community are African-American, 60 percent are over the age of 65, nearly 100 percent fall below the federal guidelines for poverty, and 80 percent are without a regular health-care provider.

Agriculture remains the major industry for the Tillery community, although a maximum-security prison farm is located there. A cafe/convenience store is open for breakfast and lunch. There is only one gas station

This material is based upon work supported by the Corporation for National Service under Learn and Serve America: Higher Education Grant No. 95-HB00006. Opinions or points of view expressed in this document are those of the authors and do not necessarily reflect the official positions of the Corporation or the Learn and Serve America program.

and one grocery store. Residents describe themselves as "hostage" to the store owners, since these businesses open when the owners feel like it and close when the owners are ready. The nearest health-care facility is 20 miles away. There is no public transportation or even taxi service. Homes are isolated and often not visible from the road. The area of the county leads the state for the number of outdoor privies still in use. For those whose image of rural North Carolina comes from Andy Griffith's television shows, Mayberry of the 1960s would have to be considered a metropolis in comparison with Tillery of the 1990s.

Halifax County is one of the state's more rural and poor counties (ranking 88 out of 100 in family income level). Tillery is one of the poorest and most isolated communities in the area, almost worthy of the description of an enclave when its socioeconomic conditions are compared with the rest of Halifax County. Standard public health and census data were of little help in getting a true picture of the health needs of the community.

Concerned Citizens of Tillery

Despite its poverty and isolation, Tillery has a strong community-based organization whose purpose is to promote and improve the social, economic, and educational welfare of its citizens through self-development of its members. This organization, Concerned Citizens of Tillery (CCT), was formed in 1978 when the county school board attempted to close the community's only school, Tillery Chapel Elementary School. From 1978 to 1981, CCT kept the school doors open, but in 1981, the school closed. That year, CCT was incorporated as a nonprofit organization and has become a model community-based organization whose philosophy is that each community needs to organize around issues most important to it. CCT strives to define community concerns positively and to convert "problems" into "issues" that can be addressed by concrete actions.

History of East Carolina University's Involvement With the Tillery Community

In 1978, the North Carolina Student Rural Health Coalition began yearly health fairs in various parts of medically underserved areas of North Carolina. Tillery was included as one of these sites because of its lack of access to health care and because of the presence of the CCT group. Over time, the health status of the community made it increasingly clear that the people of Tillery needed something more than the yearly health fairs. In an attempt to meet the community's health needs, a monthly free health clin-

elective medical students and faculty of the ECU School of Medicine was established in 1987.

The clinic was formed on and continues to operate on a community-oriented primary-care model with active input and participation by community members. Specific actions taken by community members include advertising the clinic, providing transportation to and from the clinic, making appointments, checking in patients, and arranging for referrals when indicated. Until 1989, the clinic activities were held in the community center. Medical students would set up makeshift examination rooms using egg-crate mattresses on top of dining tables and sheets for partitions. In 1989, a sweet potato curing house built during the Great Depression but subsequently abandoned was moved to a site adjacent to the community center and renovated as the present clinic building. It has been aptly named "The Curin' House" (although the emphasis is on prevention, not cure). In 1992, the Tillery community, represented by CCT and ECU, won the first international Healthier Community Award given by the Health Care Forum for successfully undertaking the best community-based initiative to improve health care.

Service-Learning in Tillery

The successes of The Curin' House and the coalition between CCT and the ECU School of Medicine led to the expansion of the university's involvement with the community via the Tillery Learn&Serve Community Project. The overall goal of the TLC was to improve access to health care for Tillery residents. For this project to be a success, the community had to be viewed as both patient and classroom. This was accomplished by a team effort, which consisted of multidisciplinary student groups and citizens of the community itself.

For some of the disciplines, viewing the community as patient was a new experience, since their focus was traditionally on individual patients with individual blends of problems. A comprehensive treatment plan was to be developed through collaboration and cooperation of all members of the student health-care delivery team. While each of the disciplines would eventually offer its particular area of expertise in the execution of the plan, the team had to form the plan working side by side on a common task with students and community members.

A community orientation program was initiated to acquaint students with Tillery. Presentations on the cultural and historical roots of the community were given within the community. Students were introduced to key members of the CCT and were invited to attend church services and join the senior citizens at their weekly lunch. Sensitivity training was conducted both on campus and within the community. Students took tours of one of the original resettlement homes, a historical plantation home, and the local prison farm.

One of the first major decisions of the project was to determine the form for the community health needs assessment. It was decided that a door-to-door survey of each household would be done with pairs of students visiting the homes. The instrument for them to use needed to be comprehensive enough to meet the intervention planning needs of the various disciplines involved with the project but manageable in length and complexity to suit the community. The Rand SF-32 questionnaire, generally used by professionals in the field, was selected as the core of the survey tool because it was a validated instrument that would provide overall community health-assessment measures.

Students and community members were invited to modify or add questions where appropriate. This activity became a learning process in itself as students and community members experienced a give-and-take deciding the wording and inclusion of various questions. For instance, the standard question on yearly income was modified to include more income ranges at the lower end of the scale. Questions on availability of indoor plumbing and access or use of well water were added along with questions on proximity to cultivated fields. Additions to physical-limitation questions included such items as "Are you able to chop wood or hang clothes on the line?" and "Are you able to walk to your mail box?" in order to more nearly reflect daily activities and tasks in this particular rural environment. Attitude and perception questions were also added to determine how the community residents viewed their interactions with the health-care community. By the time the students and community members modified, added to, and improved the survey, it had grown to 161 fixed-alternative questions.

Once the instrument and survey protocol were approved by the ECU Human Subjects Committee, the community-wide assessment began. Since all 500 households were to be approached for the survey, there was a need to inform the entire community that the students would be visiting. A kick-off event was held at the community center building with a free meal, free transportation, numerous local politicians and dignitaries, and considerable publicity. The purpose of the kickoff was to introduce the community residents to the idea of the survey and to familiarize them with the faces of at least some of the students who would be knocking on their doors.

Soon after the kickoff, students in teams of two began visiting the homes of Tillery residents for the purpose of administering the survey. While home visiting was not new to nursing students, it was a new experience for students in many of the other health disciplines. For some students, the idea of knocking on a stranger's door was frightening at first. However, the students were warmly welcomed, and only rarely did a community resident refuse to participate in the study. To the surprise of many students, the elderly residents especially enjoyed the visit and wanted to talk at length with them. An appreciation of the strength and pride of the community came through via these interactions. The students were also surprised at the advice that community residents sometimes offered them. For instance, one community health education student was recovering from bronchitis and still had a nagging cough. She was delighted with the wide range of home remedies that were recommended to her by various residents.

Students involved in the survey process found that this data-gathering role was sometimes very different from the normal student role. On the other hand, the experience was quite complementary to the student role and greatly enhanced the students' appreciation of the differences and similarities of viewing individuals as patients versus viewing the community as patient.

Elements of Service-Learning

Service-learning has been defined as "a method of education aimed at fostering an increase in a participant's capacity to contribute to the common good" (Park 1995). As noted earlier in this monograph, elements commonly identified with service-learning programs are that they (1) meet actual community needs, (2) are coordinated in collaboration with the school and community, (3) are integrated into the curriculum, (4) provide structured time for reflection, (5) provide students with opportunities to use newly acquired academic skills and knowledge in a real-life situation, (6) extend student learning beyond the classroom by enhancing what is taught, (7) help to foster the development of a sense of caring for others, and (8) encourage an ethic of citizenship (Greenberg 1995; Park 1995; Pickeral 1995). The Tillery Learn&Serve Community Project endeavored to incorporate all eight of these elements as discussed below.

1. *Meet actual community needs.* The Tillery community is active in identifying and finding solutions to its needs. There is no doubt that the community has a need for better access to health care. This project was designed to help develop a long-range plan with which the students could help the community to meet that need. Obvious barriers to health care such as geographical and social isolation, lack of transportation, high cost of care, and cultural ignorance by health-care professionals are but a few of the issues that students in cooperation with CCT attempted to address.

2. *Coordinated in collaboration with the school and community.* The ECU

School of Medicine and CCT had a long-standing relationship in working together to improve health care in the community. This project expanded on that collaboration with the inclusion of various other health professions disciplines.

3. *Integrated into the curriculum.* Initially, student involvement was elective and accomplished through students' enrolling in a special-topics independent study course within their own discipline or enrolling in the Introduction to Community Health course open to students in all disciplines and offered in the School of Health and Human Performance. Various disciplines are now integrating rotations through Tillery within their curricula.

4. *Provide structured time for reflection.* All students involved in the project were required to keep journals chronicling their before, during, and after thoughts on each interaction with the community. End-of-semester sharing seminars were held to discuss these journals. On clinic days, after the clinic closed, a reflection circle was conducted at the community center building at which community members and students shared their experiences of the day.

5. *Provide students with opportunities to use newly acquired academic skills and knowledge in a real-life situation.* East Carolina University is located in the rural eastern part of North Carolina. Despite its rural surroundings, ECU is home to a modern medical center that provides quality clinical opportunities for all students within the various health disciplines. The Tillery community was a long way from the modern medical center both physically and philosophically. Students were required to adapt to the reality of this rural enclave.

6. *Extend student learning beyond the classroom by enhancing what is taught.* Students involved in the TLC project learned much more than community assessment skills and clinical practice. Journal entries described the realization that health care did not so much depend on equipment and buildings as it did on blending sound clinical knowledge with respect and caring for clients. Students also developed a deeper understanding of the role and educational requirements of other health disciplines. Working on the common task of conducting the community needs assessment allowed students to work cooperatively without competition or comparison. Students realized that in most ways they were the same as their colleagues in different academic disciplines, and, probably more important, they realized their commonalities with the community residents in wanting security, happiness, and a sense of purpose in life.

7. *Help to foster the development of a sense of caring for others.* One of the most encouraging parts of the TLC project was observing how, on the one hand, the students developed a strong sense of caring about Tillery and its citizens while, on the other hand, the community showed a reciprocal car-

ing for and about the students. The students expressed a desire to continue to visit Tillery during their summer vacations and were anxious to see the cultivated fields at harvest time and to see whether CCT was successful in its next ambitious project — purchasing an empty plantation house.

8. *Encourage an ethic of citizenship.* The experience of working in a rural isolated community with community members who provided role models for civic pride and responsibility was literally humbling according to many students. For most, the experience gave them a sense of optimism that problems could be addressed and solved through grass-roots cooperation and collaboration.

Conclusion

The TLC project continues. Next year, students will expand the clinic hours and provide more clinical services. The Learn and Serve America grant has allowed for the purchase of much-needed equipment. Plans are being made to conduct a community-wide health awareness campaign to inform the citizens of the added services at the clinic. Each of the disciplines will begin to expand its role within the community, drawing on the results of the community needs assessment. The project to date has shown how a university can use a community as a classroom and form a partnership in which students and communities learn from each other.

References

Greenberg, J.S. (1995). "Health Care: First the Heart, Then the Head." *Journal of Health Education* 26(4): 214-223.

Park, E. (1995). Internet discussion group: *Service-Learning@csf.colorado.edu.*

Pickeral, T. (1995). Internet discussion group: *Service-Learning@csf.colorado.edu.*

Service-Learning Lessons From the Chambered Nautilus

by Evelyn D. Quigley, Betty Sayers, and Ruth Hanson

The MeritCare Health System, located in the rich farmland of the Red River valley in southeast North Dakota and southwest Minnesota, supported education and research programs early in the organization's 80-year history. Along with a growing population in the Red River valley, the need for medical clinics, hospitals, and skilled workers increased. Hospital directors recognized the importance of investing in the education of future employees and instituted a school of nursing, accredited training programs for radiology technicians and respiratory therapists, and a residency program for medical doctors.

The Fargo/Moorhead community is richly endowed with two state-supported universities, one private college, and two technical schools that offer a wide variety of training programs in the health professions. In 1976, a college president asked Evelyn Quigley, then a director of nursing at MeritCare and president of the District Nurses Association, to serve on a committee to design a curriculum for an upper-division baccalaureate degree in nursing. MeritCare leaders recognized the contributions that baccalaureate nurses could offer the organization and later phased out their diploma nursing school, thereby tying nursing education programs to the state and private colleges in the area. Partnerships between MeritCare and educational institutions were formalized in the 1970s, and since that time leaders in both academia and the health-care system serve together on boards and committees deciding policies that affect nursing education and employment.

Links Between Service-Learning and Organizational Learning

Due to the changing dynamics of the health-care business, learning at MeritCare has evolved from traditional education and skill-building programs to service-learning. It is our belief that organizations that fail to assess the needs of their customers and employees, and redesign services accordingly, are at risk.

Employees stuck in antiquated work habits and thought patterns throttle their organizations because their capacity to respond to either incremental or revolutionary change is compromised. Is it possible for groups/organizations to free themselves from their unwieldy work patterns and renew themselves? How can change be wrought among large groups of people? Can service-learning concepts stimulate organizational learning and thereby organizational change? Peter Senge (1990) and Margaret Wheatley (1992) write insightfully about organizations and change. Senge finds that successful, thriving organizations share a vision, reveal and ruthlessly critique their mental models of the world and their work, and continuously learn, adopt, and create. Wheatley applies molecular models to organizational change and concludes that, like molecules in the atmosphere, ideas form an invisible web in organizations. The web is woven out of shared beliefs, values, and mission.

Service-learning not only connects theory with application and practice but also creates an environment where both the provider of the service and the recipient learn from each other. Specifically, Senge (1990) writes, learning organizations are "organizations where people continually expand their capacity to create the results they truly desire, where new and expansive patterns of thinking are nurtured, where collective aspiration is set free, and where people are continually learning how to learn together" (3).

Fulfilling the promise of the learning organization is surely a noble task for any organization, but virtue aside, in the economic climate of managed care, the kind of learning implied by the learning organization — i.e., the kind of deliberate, reciprocal learning known as "service-learning" — is a requisite for business survival. Although health-care dollars are shrinking, support for service-learning is increasing in the MeritCare organization.

Field Theory Applied in the Organization

Small and not-so-small achievements develop service-learning into a way of life in organizations, or, as Wheatley (1992) has described it, into an "organizational field." Field theory discerns a universe that "resembles an ocean, filled with interpenetrating influences and invisible structures that connect" (51). Field theory looks beyond organizational charts, structures, and written policies to reveal the invisible world of organizational life that is a virtual web of connections. Fields are powerful organizers and influence those who penetrate them. Fields are governed by culture, vision, and values. Wheatley (1992) writes: "In a field view of organizations, clarity about values or vision is important, but it's only half the task. To create the field, the culture, vision, and values need to be disseminated widely. The field must reach all corners of the organization, involve everyone, and be available everywhere" (55). Field theory illustrates the complexity of facilitating the change from traditional learning to service-learning. New programs require leaders to examine the needs of the population, determine available resources, assess the skills required to enact the change, and educate the participants. Formal policies, unwritten rules, multitudes of relationships, and personal decisions coalesce to form a field where both the service provider and the recipient learn from each other, and one where participants engage in opportunities to explore the civic and social responsibilities of nursing education, practice, and research perspectives.

Vision and Value Statements

The medium that nourishes service-learning in MeritCare is an enduring commitment to education. In 1995, the significance of education and research was articulated in the MeritCare Health System vision statement: "To be a comprehensive health system, dedicated to a continuum of care that is quality-driven, cost-effective, and enhanced by education and research." Learning was underscored in the corporate values: "A commitment to excellence in health care, education, and research; a commitment to our customers, to our patients, and families; a commitment to support one another, recognizing and appreciating each other's talents and efforts." The MeritCare vision and values statements elevated the importance of education and research, and officially endorsed the freedom to learn, explore, invent, and change for everyone in the organization.

Application of Vision and Values

Can an organization avoid the decline of its corporate vision statements into inert, tired slogans? At MeritCare, the response is "Yes." The corporate vision and values statements were transformed from written words into lively action when money was dedicated to further the educational goals of the employees through tuition reimbursement. Currently, the organization sets aside approximately $65,000 for tuition reimbursement on a first-come, first-served basis. Continuing education is also supported by the organization with time off and some funding for conferences.

Employees enthusiastically access these opportunities to build their skill and knowledge base. Those who are fervent become advocates of service-learning as they link theory with practice at the work site. The employees, as students, enliven the shared vision and values. The organization benefits, employees benefit, and ultimately so do our customers.

MeritCare has raised and nurtured a sizable cadre of mentors. Many staff are trained as trainers to teach business management, leadership, customer service, and personal management skills within the organization because more learning needs to take place at points of service to improve how we respond to the needs of our customers. Many employees recognize the importance of their roles as teachers, collaborators, colleagues, and consultants. Their learning partners may be patients, family members, colleagues, students, or individuals in the community.

Ideally, a health system's vision statement influences nursing practice and impacts the two core elements essential to service-learning: (1) Service activities help meet community needs that the community identifies as important, and (2) educational components are structured to enhance critical thinking and reflection on the service activities and community needs.

Innovations in medical technology and drastic changes in health-care economics continue to shape the training needs of health-care professionals. Several months ago, MeritCare hosted a meeting where nursing educators at both the technical school and college/university levels could meet with their colleagues in the hospital to converse about common interests and issues. For the first time in the 15 or more years that nursing leaders and faculty have been meeting, the managers of the home-care and ambulatory-care sites were invited to attend. They fielded most of the questions because the educators were aware that more patients, and thereby more practical experiences for their students, were likely to be in the patients' homes under the care of home-health-agency nurses and clinic nurses rather than in the hospital. The business is evolving toward outpatient care, and educators need to establish new relationships, safeguards, and programs for their students' experiences. The role of leaders in the MeritCare System is to identify community needs, find the expertise in the community to ensure that support and safety systems are in place, and facilitate the change process.

A successful method to learn from and respond to our patients and our communities was instituted in 1992. The MeritCare Foundation earmarked money to fund projects identified by people in the communities served by MeritCare. A committee of foundation board members, physicians, administrators, and MeritCare employees reviews grant applications. Proposals are evaluated by the following criteria: (1) benefit to patients/families/communities, (2) benefit to MeritCare, and (3) correlation with MeritCare strategic plans and vision. Approximately $100,000 has been awarded to date. Examples of three projects that were funded in the 1995-1996 fiscal year follow:

- *Title:* Working Together — Pathways to Peace and Safety
  Service Area: MeritCare clinics in Bemidji, Bagley, Clearbrook, and Cass Lake
  Award: $7,500
  Description: A program to prevent violence was implemented in each of the service areas. Education focused on peace and safety was sponsored in the four areas. Activities included "Celebrate Kindness Week," the "Clothes-Line Project," and other community benefit/awareness programs. The project received wide community support, as evidenced by additional donations of $1,785 from the communities.

- *Title:* "Baby, Think It Over" Teen Pregnancy Prevention
  Service Area: MeritCare clinic in Mayville
  Award: $2,500
  Description: The focus of the program was to encourage teens to practice abstinence while providing them with information on choices through classroom instruction and interactive activities, including the "Think It Through Review," a play put on by students from MSU. The program also utilized lifelike battery-powered "Baby, Think It Over" dolls to demonstrate the demands of caring for an infant. This program has enjoyed a lot of media attention. Students are receptive to the information. Many students have made posters or done other projects for 4-H and other youth organizations.
- *Title:* Translation Services Training
  Service Area: Social Services
  Award: $4,781
  Description: In a collaborative effort with the Cultural Diversity Project and other community organizations, MeritCare Health System established a formal training system for professional translators. This program benefits non-English-speaking patients through improving access to quality medical services by enhancing communication. Thirty-five translators received the training.

Another recent example of service-learning that was supported by a MeritCare Foundation grant involved a MeritCare nurse, employed at the emergency center, who identified an ongoing problem. She saw the same families reporting incidents of domestic abuse returning time after time to the emergency center. She asked, "Can the emergency center staff improve the care we deliver to these families?" Due to the constraints of time, budget, and tradition, her colleagues discouraged her efforts. Despite their disparaging remarks, she pressed on with her project. Bolstered by the vision statement and MeritCare's commitment to service activities, she sought and received organizational support through an internal foundation grant. She designed a research project in which she asked the clients to define the services that were most appropriate for them, and then she wrote a curriculum to educate hospital staff, police, and other providers in the community to respond with more sensitivity to the needs of this group.

Service-Learning Leaders

In an organization that professes to value learning, leaders need to model the organization's principles. Senge (1990) writes, "Learning organizations are possible because deep down, we are all learners" (4). Effective leaders differentiate among "right" answers, rote learning, and learning environments that foster innovative thinking. Learners do not have the answers, but they are willing to examine what they are doing and investigate what may or may not work. In our organization, we expect innovators and experimenters to understand the learning process and, whenever appropriate, to approach it as a research design. We encourage research projects and often provide the means whereby the investigations and outcomes can be published and disseminated in forums at the work site and at regional, state, and national conventions.

The Spider's Offering to Service-Learning: Service-Learning in Action

An apt image for service-learning is that of a spider spinning her web. The spider spins forward, traces back, drops down, circles, and connects strands until the pattern forms. The web illustrates service-learning as being circular and responsive, in contrast to the linear and often insensitive nature of Western/academic learning modes. Karen Aylesworth, ICU manager, and Mark Papke-Larson, chaplain, articulated the web metaphor in their description of service-learning in action at North Country Regional Hospital in Bemidji, Minnesota, a 98-bed acute-care regional hospital with inpatient and outpatient rehabilitation service, hospice, home care, and dialysis.

Problem Identification

Karen manages the critical-care unit in the hospital concurrent with academic work through the University of Minnesota toward a master's degree in nursing science with a major emphasis in administration. To satisfy requirements for a nursing administration class, she was asked to study culture in the organizational setting. She was assigned a mentor in the MeritCare Health System, who shared experiences and current literature on cultural topics and introduced Karen to others in the organization who contributed additional insights. Karen recalled the "heady" mixture of theory, mentors, and talk about shared values and vision. In this experience, theory stimulated thought and inspired research that resulted in service-learning action at her workplace.

For Mark, interest in service-learning was sparked by an employee's comment following pipe ceremonies administered by Native American traditional healers for two ventilator patients in the ICU. The pipe ceremony involves, among other things, prayers and burning a small amount of tobacco in a sacred pipe. A nurse in the unit expressed her distaste for the ceremony and implied, "It is only a flashy show." The nurse's frank comments troubled Mark and alerted him to his own blind spot in understanding the values salient to the Native American population, who account for 20 percent of the patients in the health center. Mark became aware that feelings of distrust, misunderstanding, and discomfort were common among hospital staff with regard to Native American spiritual practices.

Mark expressed his concerns to Karen, who acknowledged her own lack of information about the ceremony. They agreed that a problem had surfaced, and both wanted to explore its dimensions. Their inquiries revealed misunderstandings about the healing potential of the ceremony, fears that burning tobacco in the vicinity of oxygen tanks could cause explosions, and many other questions about Native American behaviors that appeared unreasonable to the staff in the unit. Mark and Karen asked themselves, "What's going on here?" and concluded that the underlying issue was differing views about healing. The dissonance between the technical hospital culture and Native American traditions was undermining quality patient care. Instead of blaming and accusing staff for their rigid attitudes, they recognized an opportunity to turn a problem into a learning experience, and a plan evolved.

Process for Stimulating Cultural Learning

The first priority was to arrange an environment in which the care givers would feel comfortable and receptive to new ideas. Karen and Mark focused on two questions: "Where do critical-care staff feel secure enough to reveal their concerns?" "What are the links between modern medical practice and Native American healing ceremonies?" They concluded that the most comfortable place for employees to inquire and learn was in their own ICU staff meetings, and that the ideal link might be to focus on patient care.

The next step was locating a credible, knowledgeable person to facilitate the experience. According to folk wisdom in the realm of spiritual teaching, "When the student is ready, the teacher will appear." Karen and Mark became aware of a wise individual who offered experience and insight into both the culture of the health-care setting and the Native American culture.

In the staff meeting, the cultural consultant opened his talk with words of praise and thanks directed toward the ICU staff for their excellent work in the unit caring for the Native American people. He identified himself as a cultural bridge and explained that in a multicultural world, people and institutions often need to bridge different beliefs, values, and ways of doing things. The staff realized that hospitals always span cultures, and that medical professionals, unlike many other professionals, need to be connectors between differing worldviews because of the intimacy inherent in patient care. He related to his audience through story telling. The stories illustrated the various ways healing occurs in different cultures and the importance for both staff and patient to feel comfortable with a variety of modalities. He suggested that when people understand each other and feel secure in their relationship, respect is established and patient care improves. The staff listened attentively. They asked questions and openly expressed their personal fears and beliefs.

Karen suggested that a test for comfort with cultural practices is the ability of a nurse to say to a patient or family member, "I know I'm going to make mistakes. Will you correct me? I want to learn." Mark said, "I believe that, basically, medical staff want to provide healing, but that, due to their history and training, managing technology is usually their priority. The healing needs of the individual, the family, the community, as well as of themselves may not be addressed." Karen agreed, saying, "Nursing professionals talk about mind, body, and spirit as if they were three distinct entities, when in many cultures, they are one."

Outcomes

In evaluating the experience, Karen reported that staff were speaking to the families directly rather than following their former practice of asking her, as manager, to solve problems. In fact, she has not been asked to intervene with a Native American family since the dialogue occurred. Woven in shift reports were mentions of eagle feathers and other Native American customs. The changes among the staff were subtle, but present. Mark said, "Something happened as a result of the intervention — fewer judgmental statements and more examples of nurses' validating the ceremonies and the family beliefs." A written policy on spiritual care and procedures relating to American Indian cultural and religious practices evolved. (The policy is reproduced at the end of this chapter.)

Facilitated dialogue sessions on Native American spiritual practices are now arranged for other groups of patient-care providers in the system upon their request. To date, several different work groups have participated in the learning experience.

When Karen and Mark reflect on the process and outcomes of service-learning in the health system, they acknowledge that many issues remain unrecognized and unresolved, and that staff may circle back to old behaviors, but fashioning a web of mutual respect is under way. In essence, Mark and Karen thoughtfully organized an environment where both the provider of the service and the recipient learn from each other. Their work provides a framework to guide institutions in efforts to collaborate with consumers and explore the civic and social responsibilities of nursing education, practice, and research.

Summary

In revolutionary times, achievements in service-learning may fall victim to the speed of change and the spread of events. Evelyn Quigley, MeritCare vice president, has said:

> When I fathom the sea of change churning the health-care business and realize that some individuals and populations in our community struggle to obtain the services they need, I retain some level of comfort by gazing at an artist's drawing of the chambered nautilus seashell that hangs on my office wall. A cross-section of the spiral shell reveals incremental but steady increases in the capacity of each new chamber to house the growing nautilus organism.
>
> The following lines from the poem "The Chambered Nautilus," written by Oliver Wendell Holmes (1808-1894), remind me that great tasks are accomplished with patience over time by a series of small acts.
>
> Year after year beheld the silent toil
> > That spread his lustrous coil;
> > Still, as the spiral grew,
> He left the past year's dwelling for the new,
> Stole with soft step its shining archway through,
> > Built up its idle door,
> Stretched in his last-found home, and knew the old no more.

The chambered nautilus offers a final lesson on cultivating a shared learning environment as he "left the past year's dwelling for the new" and "knew the old no more." Organizations that champion service-learning programs replace the narrow and often costly autonomous models of the past with teaching-learning models that involve clients' and providers' working in partnership to codesign plans of care. Service-learning leaders, who design ways to integrate health-care services with community programs, minimize duplication and collaborate with their customers and other providers to advance a global vision of healthier communities.

References

Senge, P. (1990). *The Fifth Discipline*. New York, NY: Doubleday Currency.

Wheatley, M.J. (1992). *Leadership and the New Science*. San Francisco, CA: Berrett-Koehler.

Spiritual Care and Procedures
Relating to American Indian Cultural and Religious Practices

Purpose of Procedures.
In keeping with our mission of providing excellent health care, North Country Health Services is dedicated to ensuring that patients and families receive respectful, fair treatment in the practice of cultural and religious beliefs. As a health-care organization serving the American Indian population, we will be responsive to the specific request made for religious services from patients and families.

Sacred Ceremonies.
On occasion, a Spiritual Advisor is called by an American Indian patient or family to conduct a healing spiritual ceremony. This ceremony might include large numbers of extended family members. If the number of family members is hampering care of the patient, restrictions can be discussed among the family and staff. The chapel on the fourth floor of the hospital could also be used as a place to have the ceremonies.

Sacred herbs such as sweet grass, sage, cedar, and tobacco may be burned by the patient, family, or Spiritual Advisor in very small quantities, possibly in a pipe or incense burner. While these practices are being performed, they should not be interrupted unless the practice endangers others. The resolution of any problems in regard to these practices should be carried out with respect and consideration of the patient's right and hospital rules and regulations. Clinical judgment is required, and each situation must be approached looking to the particular needs of the patient/family.

Safety Issues Related to Oxygen Usage.
1. Turn off oxygen for the length of the ceremony if possible. An oxygen saturation of 85 percent to 90 percent is recommended as a minimum. If saturation falls below this, oxygen must be resumed. Good clinical judgment is required.

2. Respectfully alert the individual performing the ceremony of the need for caution regarding oxygen and a heat source.

3. If oxygen cannot be disconnected, a safety distance of five feet should be maintained between the oxygen-delivery device and the heat source. Respectfully ask the individual performing the ceremony to keep the heat source as far from the oxygen-delivery device as possible. Good clinical judgment is required.

Sacred Objects.
American Indian cultural and religious practices include sacred objects as well as ceremonies that sometimes include a Spiritual Advisor (sometimes called a Medicine Man). Eagle feathers, tobacco ties, pipes, beaded articles, and leather pouches are considered sacred objects to many American Indian people. As health-care workers (non-Indian), we may not fully understand the significance of these objects in relationship to the patient and family's spiritual/physical healing. Therefore, any and all sacred objects should not be moved or touched without permission of the patient or a family member.

Organ Donation.
Some American Indian people believe a body should be buried with all body parts intact. Asking an Indian family about a possible organ donation could be a delicate matter.

Resources.
Contact the hospital Chaplain, Clinical Supervisor, or Social Services to provide support and help in addressing specific clinical situations if necessary.

Materials From
Service-Learning as a Pedagogy in Nursing

by Elaine Cohen, Susan Johnson, Lois Nelson, and Connie Peterson

Contents

Syllabus (edited for publication)

Service-Learning Assignment

Student Project Final Report: "Caring in the Community"

TRI-COLLEGE UNIVERSITY NURSING CONSORTIUM/
CONCORDIA COLLEGE AND NORTH DAKOTA STATE UNIVERSITY

NURSING 351, Nursing Concepts

CREDITS: 1 Course (75% theory; 25% clinical component)

PREREQUISITES: Nursing 341 and 361

TIME: Monday, Wednesday 8:30 am - 9:40 am; Friday 8:00 am - 9:10 am
                  Clinical Component as arranged

FACULTY: Susan Johnson, Coordinator, and Connie Peterson

REQUIRED TEXTBOOKS:
Beare, P. G. and Myers, J. L. (1994). *Principles and practices of adult health nursing.* St. Louis: C.V. Mosby Co.
Dickason, E. J. et al. (1994). *Maternal-infant nursing care.* St. Louis: C.V. Mosby Co.
Potter, P. and Perry, A. (1993). *Fundamentals of nursing.* St. Louis: C.V. Mosby Co. (Text and Study Guide).

COURSE DESCRIPTION:
Focuses on application of the nursing process to selected, common disorders of the adult client.

COURSE OBJECTIVES:
1.   Expand awareness of ethical concerns in selected nursing situations.
2.   Identify strategies to promote health for a variety of common healthcare situations.
3.   Identify and value caring behaviors in a variety of healthcare situations.
4.   Identify therapeutic nursing interventions for culturally and socially diverse persons experiencing (or at risk of experiencing) an altered health state.

TEACHING METHODOLOGY:
Teaching methods will include lecture, discussion, audio-visual aids, worksheets, and a service learning project.

INSTRUCTOR EXPECTATIONS:
1.   Class attendance is highly encouraged. Attendance for "College Laboratory" is required. Students may be excused from class or laboratory under certain circumstances (family crisis, college-sanctioned activities, illness). If this occurs the student is expected to notify the instructor prior to the absence if at all possible. Make-up assignments may be required for absences. It is the student's responsibility to initiate this inquiry. Make-up tests must be re-scheduled with the instructor on the first day back. Students taking more than one exam late, except in the case of unusual circumstances, will lose 10 points.
2.   Because of the nature of the profession of nursing, students are expected to conduct themselves in the classroom and clinical settings with academic honesty, integrity, and in an ethical manner. Failure to demonstrate this kind of behavior may result in disciplinary action, including failure in the course or on an assignment, academic warning, probation, and/or suspension from the program or the college/university.
3.   Safety and confidentiality of the client must be maintained at all times. Unsafe or inappropriate behavior can result in failure of the course.
4.   Students may earn credit for this course by challenge examination. Details for course challenge are in the Nursing Student Handbook.
Any student with disabilities who requires special accommodations in this course are invited to share these concerns or requests as soon as possible with the instructor.

COURSE EVALUATION WILL BE BASED ON THE FOLLOWING:
    4 Exams
    1 Final Exam
    Service Project Assignments - Refer to "Service-Learning (SL) Assignment"
    Service Project Hours (P/F)

Course Outline	Learning Activities
A. Spiritual Health and the Nursing Process 1. Definition of spirituality 2. What are spiritual needs? 3. Spiritual needs assessment 4. Nursing diagnosis: Spiritual Distress 5. Spiritual care *This content relates to the Service-Learning site - Hospice*	**Required Readings:** Potter & Perry, Chapter 33. Do study guide pp. 138-139. 1. Discuss relationship of spiritual health to physiological and psychosocial health. 2. Assess components of spiritual health and identify signs of unmet spiritual needs. 3. List interventions for spiritual care.
B. College Lab 1 - Parish Nursing Role *This content relates to the Service-Learning site - Parish Nursing Program*	**Required Readings:** Beal, G. (1994). "The parish as a healing place." *Bond*, Winter Issue, 4-6. (In lab) Ratzloff, T. (1993). "A calling and pastor/nurse serves parish from cradle to grave." *Minnesota Nurse*, 6(1), 6-9. (In lab) Parish Nurse Brochures - (In class) 1. Discuss the role of the Parish Nurse.
C. Integrating Social-Cultural Aspects into Nursing Care 1. Definitions of terms 2. Nursing principles related to transcultural nursing 3. Common sociocultural characteristics *This content relates to the Service-Learning site - Refugee Resettlement Program, Retirement Center, Homeless Shelters, Indian Health Center*	**Required Readings:** Potter & Perry, Chapter 4. 1. Examine and clarify personal sociocultural beliefs that may influence interactions with clients. 2. Describe the relationship of sociocultural background to health and illness beliefs and practices. 3. Compare concepts of traditional and modern health and illness beliefs and practices. 4. Discuss ways in which planning and implementing nursing interventions can be adapted to the client's ethnicity.
D. Surgery - Nursing Care in the Preoperative Phase 1. Assessment 2. Client preparation and support 3. Informed consent	**Required Readings:** Potter 1600-1630. Optional: Beare, Chapter 22. 1. List factors to include in the preoperative assessment of a surgical client. 2. Discuss and demonstrate preparation for surgery and appropriate client teaching.
E. Surgery - Nursing Care in the Intraoperative Phase 1. Types of anesthesia 2. Ethical/legal aspects of surgery 3. Safety aspects of nursing care 4. Terminology related to surgery	**Required Readings:** Beare, Chapter 23. 1. Compare and contrast the actions and side effects of general, regional, and local anesthesia. 2. Identify common threats to the safety of the surgical client. 3. Identify legal/ethical issues in the surgical setting.
F. College Lab 2 - Clinical Skills for Surgical Nursing 1. Surgical team 2. Microbes and surgical aseptic technique 3. Professional resources: AORN	**Required Readings:** Beare, Chapter 23. **Watch Video Before Class:** *Fundamentals of Aseptic Technique.* 1. Describe the roles of the surgical team members. 2. Recognize breaks in aseptic technique. 3. Appreciate the importance of surgical asepsis. 4. Describe the purposes of AORN.

G. Surgery - Nursing Care in the Postoperative Phase 1. Assessment in PACU 2. Common post-anesthesia problems and related nursing care 3. Nursing activities to promote recovery	**Required Readings:** Potter & Perry, pp. 1635-1647. Optional: Beare, Chapter 24. 1. Discuss physiological disruptions that occur as a result of surgery. 2. Discuss the nursing process for clients in the postoperative phase.
H. Sleep 1. Rest 2. Sleep -- Kinds of sleep 3. Assessment of rest/sleep need 4. Common sleep disorders 5. Sleep deprivation	**Required Readings:** Potter & Perry, pp. 1144-1173. Beare, pp. 383-389. 1. Differentiate between REM and NREM sleep cycle patterns. 2. Identify clinical signs and symptoms indicative of insufficient rest or sleep. 3. Identify clients that are at risk for sleep pattern disturbances and plan nursing interventions that promote rest and sleep in these clients. 4. Plan nursing interventions to limit and/or prevent sleep deprivation.
I. Nursing Care of clients with Gastrointestinal Disorders 1. Assessment of gastrointestinal function and common diagnostic tests 2. Disorders affecting the gastrointestinal system 3. Nursing process: Client with gastrointestinal disorder	**Required Readings:** Beare, Chapters 63-67. 1. Identify the etiology and pathophysiology of the gastrointestinal disorders. 2. Relate the clinical manifestations of the gastrointestinal disorders to the underlying pathophysiology. 3. Explain common laboratory diagnostic tests used to identify alterations in gastrointestinal function. 4. Apply the nursing process to clients experiencing common disorders of the gastrointestinal system. 5. Discuss primary prevention of gastrointestinal disorders.
J. College Lab 3 - Enterostomy Therapy	1. Identify the components of basic colostomy care including bag application and irrigation. 2. Identify pertinent assessment data related to the client with an ostomy. 3. Incorporate information related to ostomy care for appropriate client teaching.

K. Nursing Care of Clients with Musculoskeletal System Disorders
1. Common diagnostic tests related to musculoskeletal function
2. Disorders affecting the musculoskeletal system
    a. Traumatic injury
    b. Acquired disorders
    c. Neoplasia
3. Nursing process: Client with a musculoskeletal disorder
	Required Readings: Beare, Chapters 56, 57, 58.
	1. Identify the etiology and pathophysiology of inflammatory, acquired and neoplastic musculoskeletal disorders.
	2. Relate clinical manifestations of these disorders to the underlying pathophysiology.
	3. Identify the etiology and pathophysiology of traumatic and structural musculoskeletal disorders.
	4. Relate clinical manifestations of these disorders to the underlying pathophysiology.
	5. Apply the nursing process for clients experiencing common musculoskeletal disorders.
	6. Discuss primary prevention of musculoskeletal disorder.

L. College Lab 4 - Impact of Chronic Illness on Clients and Families *This content refers to the Service-Learning site - the Retirement Center*	**Required Readings:** Potter & Perry, Chapters 55-59. 1. Discuss the impact on the individual and family when chronic illness occurs. 2. Identify community resources and health promotion strategies to assist in chronic illness.

Page 3

M. Caring for Clients with Reproductive Disorders 1. Assessment and diagnostic testing 2. Altered reproductive functions 3. Nursing interventions for common reproductive disorders	**Required Readings:** Beare, Chapters 68, 70, 71. 1. Identify the etiology and pathophysiology of common alterations in the reproductive function. 2. Relate clinical manifestations of reproductive dysfunctions to the underlying pathophysiology. 3. apply the nursing process to clients experiencing common dysfunctions of the reproductive system. 4. Discuss primary prevention of reproductive disorders.
N. Coping with Breast Cancer 1. Common concerns of clients with breast cancer 2. Resources to promote coping	**Required Readings:** Brochures and TBA. 1. Discuss the effect of breast cancer on communication, intimacy and sexuality. 2. Discuss resources for women who have had mastectomies.
O. Caring for Clients with Infertility 1. Components of fertility 2. Tests for infertility 3. Methods of infertility management 4. Adoption	**Required Readings:** Dickason, Chapter 6. **Video:** *Infertility - Nature's Heartache* 1. Identify common causes of infertility and primary methods of diagnosis and treatment. 2. Discuss the psychosocial effects on couples experiencing the problem of infertility. 3. Discuss the nurse's role in supporting clients through diagnosis and treatment for infertility and in helping clients cope with the loss of fertility.
P. Nursing and Genetics 1. Categories of genetic diseases 2. Genetic engineering/treatment 3. Genetic counseling	**Required Readings:** Dickason, Chapter 27. 1. Describe how an individual's genetic make-up might be the basis for a disorder. 2. Enumerate the categories of genetic disorders. 3. Discuss how genetic engineering is emerging as a biological break-through. 4. Identify the nurse's role in intervention with families at risk for genetic disorders.
Q. College Lab 6 - Ethics 1. Professional ethics/values and decision making *This content refers to all sites for Service-Learning*	**Required Readings:** Potter & Perry, Chapter 13. 1. Define terms associated with ethics in nursing practice. 2. Discuss the influence of ethics on nursing practice. 3. Discuss the influence of personal and professional values on ethical decisions. 4. Review the purposes of a professional code of ethics. 5. Discuss examples of ethical conflicts confronted by nurses. 6. Discuss and apply to a case study the process used to resolve ethical problems.
R. College Lab 7 Part 1: Advanced Directives Part 2: Service Learning	**Required Readings:** Beare, p. 424. 1. Identify what "advance directives" are and ways to facilitate discussion with clients about these decisions. 2. Share concerns that have emerged from clinical projects. 3. Collaborate with group to plan presentation.
S. Caring for Clients with AIDS 1. Epidemiology 2. Effect on the Immune System 3. Clinical manifestations 4. Nursing process for the client with AIDS	**Required Readings:** Potter & Perry, Chapter 18. Beare, Chapter 40. 1. Identify high risk behaviors for contracting AIDS. 2. Describe the effect of AIDS on the immune system. 3. Explain why HIV infection is difficult to cure.

	4. Identify symptoms which may indicate HIV infection. 5. Discuss nursing care for the client with AIDS.
T. College Lab 8 - Death and Dying 1. Nursing care for the dying 2. Hospice care 3. Postmortem care *This content relates to the Service-Learning site - Hospice*	**Required Readings:** Potter & Perry, pp. 872-881. 1. Identify and discuss the role of the nurse in the care of the dying client and his/her family. 2. Become familiar with the concepts essential to hospice nursing. 3. Identify and discuss the role of the nurse in postmortem care of the deceased client.

U. Caring for Clients with Integumentary Disorders
1. Disorders affecting the integumentary system
   a. Hereditary
   b. Acquired
   c. Neoplasia
	Required Readings: Beare, Chapters 73-74.
	1. Identify the etiology and pathophysiology of common integumentary disorders in the adult client.
	2. Describe significant clinical manifestations of skin disorders as they relate to underlying pathophysiology in the adult client.
	3. Utilize the nursing process to formulate understanding of the care of the adult client with integumentary disorders.
	4. Discuss primary prevention related to care of the skin.

V. Caring for Clients with Disorders of the Hematopoietic System
1. Assessment of the hematopoietic function
2. Disorders affecting the hematopoietic system:
   a. Acquired disorders
   b. Neoplastic disorders
3. Nursing process: Client with hematopoietic disorders
	Required Readings: Beare, Chapters 37, 38, 40.
	1. Identify the etiology and pathophysiology of the common hematopoietic disorders.
	2. Relate the clinical manifestations of hematopoietic disorders to the underlying pathophysiology.
	3. Explain common laboratory diagnostic tests used to identify alterations in hematopoietic function.
	4. Apply the nursing process to clients experiencing common hematopoietic disorders.
	5. Discuss methods of primary prevention for hematopoietic disease.

W. Caring for Clients with Disorders of the Senses 1. Assessment of the Sensory System 2. Sensory Overload 3. Sensory Deprivation 4. Disorders affecting the special senses 5. Nursing process: Client with sensory disorder	**Required Readings:** Beare, Chapters 52-55, 17. 1. Identify the etiology and pathophysiology of selected sensory disorders. 2. Relate the clinical manifestations of sensory disorders to the underlying pathophysiology. 3. Apply the nursing process to clients experiencing common disorders of vision, hearing, and equilibrium 4. Discuss primary prevention related to disorders of the special senses.
X. College Lab 9 - Substance Abuse 1. Drugs and substances 2. Signs and symptoms of substance abuse 3. Nursing process for chemically dependant clients	**Required Readings:** Potter & Perry, Chapter 46. 1. Identify common drugs and substances abused and their effects on health. 2. Describe signs and symptoms of substance abuse. 3. Discuss nursing interventions for chemically dependent clients.
Y. College Lab 10, 11, 12 - Group Presentation of Clinical Projects (Service-Learning)	1. Demonstrate application and synthesis of course theory to clinical projects.

Page 5

SERVICE-LEARNING (SL) ASSIGNMENT

Description:
The overall goal of the SL project is to provide you with an unique opportunity to further develop your role as a responsible and effective citizen in the context of professional nursing. As you provide service to an agency or program you will develop your own skills and apply and integrate course theory content in meaningful ways in the community. It will provide you with a broader vision of health care. A key piece of your learning will be the reflection and structured assignments that are based on your concrete experience as well as the sharing of experiences with your peers. The SL project enhances the mission of the nursing program which is to "serve as a nursing resource to society."

Objectives for the SL Project:
1.   Appreciate the inherent values and benefits of service as part of effective citizenship.
2.   Appreciate the potential roles of nursing in the community setting in order to serve as a nursing resource for society.
3.   Apply new course content as well as previous learning to clients outside of the acute care setting.
4.   Develop greater initiative and confidence in yourself in a professional role.

Specific objectives especially for #2-4 will vary somewhat depending on the SL site. Hence, students will share their learning experience with the class, so that peers can learn from each other's experiences.

SL Project Sites (partial list):
▸   Diabetic screening project
▸   Community Outreach (YWCA Women's Shelter, New Life Center, Churches United, Good Medicine Indian Health Center)
▸   Lutheran Social Services - Refugee Resettlement Program
▸   Churches
▸   Hospice
▸   Retirement Centers

Expectations of Students:
1.   A minimum of 20 hours of service activity is expected. You will be asked to keep a log of your hours.
2.   Contact your SL site supervisor immediately to schedule an appointment to discuss your SL project objectives and the ways (roles) in which you will serve the agency to meet those objectives. You will also need a brief orientation to the facility or program so you can understand the context of your SL role in the wider organization. Refer to the guidelines in the syllabus for "Preparation for Service Paper." Take along the form "Student Service Learning Project Agreement." Complete the form and have your supervisor sign it as well as yourself. Turn it in to me and I will photocopy it. I will retain a copy and the other copy must be given to your SL supervisor.
3.   Please follow the usual expectations for clinical laboratory. Being on time, dressing in an appropriate manner, calling in if you are ill or have a true emergency, maintaining confidentiality of clients, etc. You are representing our nursing program.
4.   If you are unclear about your tasks/roles, please clarify these concerns with your SL supervisor.
5.   Make entries in your Participant/Observer Journal as soon as possible after completing your work on a given day.

Student Assignments:

1.   Service Learning Paper

Include the following components in your paper

- The reason you chose this agency.
- The mission and goals of the agency/program. (Include how this agency is funded, whether it is part of national organization; how does it promote health?)
- Description of the population served. (Are there any issues/problems the clients face on a day to day basis?)
- Personal learning objectives and activities at the agency to meet the objectives.
- Information/preparation required to prepare for effective engagement in SL project. (Readings from agency, library, text)
- Brief summary of two sources of information and/or preparation. (Be sure to include a full citation of the source.) One source should be a nursing journal article.

This paper must be typed, using APA style. Turn the paper in to me in a folder. [SL folder] It is due prior to your beginning hours of service.

2.   Personal Journal

These should be included in the SL folder mentioned above. Following each experience a journal entry should be made. (They may be handwritten) The following format should be used:

- List date and hours worked
- Describe in objective terms what you did
- Link the experience to course material (Discuss connections between course theory/objectives and what you observed or performed.)
- Reflect on your role development. (Describe your own personal reactions. What knowledge or skills did you acquire or were reinforced? What did you learn about yourself?)

**Be sure you address all of the above in your entries and especially make clear connections to theoretical concepts in Nursing 351 and as appropriate, previous courses.

3.   Final Report on Service Learning Project

Review your preparation paper and journal entries as a way to initiate your reflections on the entire project. Give your report a title; use APA style.

Components of summary:

- Name of agency, your objectives and service activities.
- What concepts from Nursing 351 can you relate to your experience?
- What knowledge or skills did you acquire from the experience?
- Discuss how ideas which you brought to the experience concerning the type of agency/ program, services, or population changed during the course.
- What did you learn about yourself?

- Discuss what you see as possible nursing roles for health promotion, research, or identification of clients with health care needs in you SL site or one similar to it.
- How could this site have been a better learning experience for you? Likewise, how might you have enhanced your own learning experience?

This must be typed and is due [date]. Include it in your SL folder.

4.   Oral Group Presentations

Students in similar agencies will be grouped together to creatively present to the rest of the class highlights of significant learning experiences as the result of the SL projects. May use role play, overheads, drawings, whatever to convey and involve your classmates with the content. Each group should plan about 10-15 minutes and then allow a couple more minutes for questions. The group will be graded as a whole.

Evaluation

Preparation paper	= 20 points
Summary paper	= 20 points
Journal entries	= 15 points
Oral Presentation	= Pass/Fail

"Caring in the Community"

by
Amy Magedanz
Junior Nursing Student, Concordia College, Moorhead, Minnesota

Community health in the Fargo-Moorhead is made of many components. Not only does it involve different agencies, but it also involves different types of caring. However, there is a common goal: to care for the homeless in the area with community resources and medical assistance.

I worked with three of these branches: The New Life Center, Salvation Army Clinic, and the Good Medicine Clinic. These centers are off-shoots of the Health Services Center. Each experience provided new ideas and information which I described in my journals. I enjoyed each situation and am glad I was able to participate.

I entered the service learning project intending to broaden my horizons, learn and solidify skills, explore different populations, and challenge myself. I did not have the opportunity to practice skills but I was able to meet my other objectives. My primary activity was observation. I shadowed two excellent nurses in three clinic settings. I helped out with an occasional blood pressure reading, pulse or temperature, but most cases did not require assessment. My job was to listen and learn.

My idea of how the clinic flowed was a little askew. I thought most of the clients were regular to the clinics and resided in the Fargo-Moorhead shelters or on the streets. I did not realize the homeless population goes through much fluctuation and changes daily. This fact makes sense, but I had to be faced with it before I understood.

I also thought the clients would come in, eager to improve their total health. I discovered they have more on their minds than holistic health care. My idea of the nursing role in this setting had to be adjusted. I thought the most important part of community nursing should be education. When the clients came in the door, they would be completely assessed and then educated on how to improve their life with proper nutrition and community assistance programs. I found out the clients had a different agenda.

Most of the clients come to the clinics for a specific reason. The clinic must meet that need first, before addressing the rest of the person. If the need is met then trust develops and the chance of the person returning for another appointment increases. If the client returns then the nurse has an open door to create continuous health assistance and serve the whole person.

The development of health service continuity may help form client history. Most of the clientele do not have a regular health provider which limits the personal medical history system as we know it. Personal medical history provides valuable information for future health care and reference. Unfortunately, this population is a hard one to put on file because of the migration factor and temporary living arrangements brought on by financial situation. So, if some trust and history can be gained, the provider's ability to serve is strengthened.

This change in my ideas made me pay close attention to the nurses and how they functioned. I noticed both nurses used a relaxed method to address the client. Both remained calm throughout the sessions and maintained eye contact. They were also not afraid to show their personal side. This was displayed by identifying with the client somehow.

The chief complaint of the individual directed the appointment and the type of assessment performed. The examination and interview appeared to involve only the affected systems, but I know the nurse was looking for

1

anything unusual. If, during this limited assessment, a significant problem other than the complaint was found, it would be addressed. The nurse would then make a referral or give appropriate medication. The process is quick and smooth. Unfortunately, it still lacks a continuous health care plan.

I learned confidence, control, and knowledge are an important part of nursing. As much as I hate to say it, some people of this population would manipulate a nurse to get items a nurse is not authorized to distribute. Even if the nurse feels comfortable and relaxed, she must remember her professional role and act accordingly.

I came face-to-face with many of the mental health and alcohol abuse problems with which the homeless struggle. The majority of the adults I contacted eith. r had a history or present problem with them. A few times I witnessed a nurse dealing with a client who was intoxicated. Community nurses must be prepared to manage situations like these.

The limited contact I did have, helped me to learn valuable things about myself. I discovered that I must have patience with my inexperience. Many times I was frustrated because I couldn't think of something to say to an individual. I was not comfortable addressing sensitive issues. I realized comfort level will come with time. It won't be any easier but I will be able to do it.

Characteristics of a therapeutic nurse include humor, sensitivity, and being non-judgmental. Learning these attributes from a book or case is not equal to applying them in practice. Fortunately, I followed two nurses bearing these qualities.

Of the three, being non-judgmental seems the most important to me. The client has come for health service, not a lecture. It is too easy to blame the person for their situation which is wrong. The nurses were open-minded and focused on the health need which helped to avoid judgment.
Another issue in nursing is differentiating between sympathy and pity. I can't think of anyone who wants to be pitied. It was amazing how the nurses were able to ask questions, be concerned, and find a way to address problems without expressing pity. I need to learn how to convey concern without pity. If I don't, I may be overcome by the reality of the situations and become depressed.

Health promotion is a nursing role which is present in almost every health facility. Health promotion is small in this setting, but it does exist. It is possible to educate some of the regulars about preventative measures and monitor their health. Some clients I encountered were involved in checking their blood pressure. Others come in regularly to get vitamins. The nurses attempt to incorporate health promotion whenever possible, but as explained earlier, it is difficult.

I gained much from this experience. Unfortunately, it is hard to capture the rewards in words, however, I do know I could have gained more. Every experience has more to offer than what is exercised. I had few opportunities to assess clients or interview them. A way to enhance my experience would have been to participate in a screening session. Unfortunately, my schedule did not allow this.

I am pleased with what I learned. The experience revealed things about people and community health I had not considered. I know I will have time to develop my skill level as I continue nursing. I appreciate the time spent with the nurses and all the answers they gave. This was a valuable lesson in the nursing art of caring.

2

Materials From
Case Study of a Service-Learning Project in a Nurse-Managed Clinic for Homeless and Indigent Individuals

by Carol L. Macnee, Deborah H. White, and Jean C. Hemphill

Contents

SYLLABUS

HDAL 1020: INTRODUCTION TO COMMUNITY SERVICE
Fall Term, 1996

Instructor: Joyce Duncan
(423) 439-5675
(423) 439-4314
(423) 926-0056
E-mail: duncanj@etsu.etsu-tn.edu

Office: Burleson Hall, 101-C and Student Activities (Culp Ctr)
Office Hours: TBA

Purpose/Course Objectives:

▸ To demonstrate community needs in Northeast Tennessee

▸ To focus on those needs in the areas of: education, the environment, health care, hunger and homelessness, and public safety, especially domestic violence

▸ To become aware of the community change process and how the student can aid in effecting that change

▸ To provide an experiential learning situation for the student through hands-on contact with agencies that deal with those issues

Texts and Requirements:
Lappe, Francis, and Paul Dubois. *The Quickening of America.* San Francisco: Jossey-Bass, Inc., 1994.
A small notebook suitable for journal entries.
There is no prerequisite for the course.

Content of Course:

Aug 26:	Introduction and pretest. *Assignment:* Ch 1
Aug 28:	Discussion of Ch 1. *Assignment:* Ch 2
Aug 30:	Discussion of Ch 2. Journal keeping
Sep 2:	Holiday
Sep 4:	Role playing exercise. *Assignment:* Ch 3
Sep 6:	Discussion of Ch 3. Trust-building exercises
Sep 9, 11, 13:	Presentations by area agencies
Sep 16:	Students will match skills with agency and select placement. *Assignment:* Ch 4
Sep 18:	Discussion of Ch 4. Multiculturalism and role play. *Assignment:* Ch 5
Sep 20:	Discussion of Ch 5. Creation of "confidentiality contract." *Assignment:* first 3-page paper (due 10/14), and Ch 6
Sep 23:	Reflections
Sep 25:	Leadership Transcript
Sep 27:	OFF
Sep 30:	Discussion of Ch 6. Letter to Editor
Oct 2:	Reflections. *Assignment:* Ch 7
Oct 4:	Discussion of Ch 7. *Assignment:* Ch 8

Oct 7:	Journal Due. "What Every Literate American Should Know"
Oct 9:	Reflections
Oct 11:	Discussion of Ch 8. Documentary Film: "Books Under Fire"
Oct 14:	Reflections. *Assignment:* Ch 9
Oct 16:	Discussion of Ch 9. *Assignment:* second 3-page paper (due 10/30), and Ch 10
Oct 18:	Discussion of Ch 10
Oct 21:	Reflections
Oct 23, 25:	OFF
Oct 28:	Film "With Honors"
Oct 30:	Film "With Honors." Paper Due
Nov 1:	Film "With Honors," discussion and reflection
Nov 4:	Reflections/Trial. *Assignment:* Chs 11 and 12
Nov 6:	Discussion of Chs 11 and 12. *Assignment:* Ch 13
Nov 8:	Journal Due. Discussion of Ch 13
Nov 11, 13, 15, 18:	Student Presentations
Nov 20:	Homelessness Game
Nov 22:	Group Presentations
Nov 25:	OFF
Nov 27:	OFF
Nov 29:	HOLIDAY
Dec 2, 4:	Group Presentations
Dec 6:	Review and Post Test

Grades Will Be Determined as Follows:

Attendance and Participation	5%
Paper I	10%
Paper II	10%
Service Hours/Agency Evaluation	20%
(30 hours hands-on, out of class)	
Journal	10%
Leadership Transcript	5%
Regional Reflections Meeting	10%
Individual Presentation	10%
Group Presentation	10%
Final Exam	10%

**** Since attendance is necessary for the success of the class and for the success of the student in the class, more than 9 absences (excused or unexcused) shall constitute automatic failure in the class. Roll will be taken daily.

** University grading scale of + and - will apply as will all university rules on conduct and plagiarism.

3

<u>The Student Will Be Required:</u>

- To complete *The Quickening of America.* Quizzes may be given.
- To read one other work which pertains to the course. Books are available from the instructor or from the library with instructor approval.
- To submit all forms promptly.
- To submit papers and presentations when they are due with the awareness that grades will be dropped for late papers or rescheduled presentations (one class period's grace, then one letter grade per class period).
- To maintain a reflections journal and to make an entry at least 3 times per week.
- To complete 30 hours of service in their placement. All else being equal, grades will be given on a sliding scale: 30 hours-A, 29-27 hours-B, 26-24 hours-C, 23-21 hours-D, 20 or less-F (equals 20 percent of total grade for class).
- To inform the instructor if there is any difficulty with the placement.
- To attend and to participate in each class.

** The student may also feel free to contact Debbie White, Director, Northeast Tennessee Consortium for Service-Learning, at the Student Activities Office in the Culp Center (#5675) or Mary Stakias (282-0800 or 323-3191), Site Placement Coordinator.

EAST TENNESSEE STATE UNIVERSITY SCHOOL OF NURSING
DEPARTMENT OF FAMILY/COMMUNITY NURSING
Spring, 1996

COURSE: FCNU 4211 - Community Health Nursing Practicum

FACULTY: Carol L. Macnee, R.N., Ph.D. (Coordinator), Yoakley Hall, Rm. 212,
                  439-7144
                  Sonda Oppewal, R.N., Ph.D., Yoakley Hall, Rm. 108, 439-6784
                  Mary Kay Anderson, R.N., Ph.D., Yoakley Hall, Rm. 210 439-7169
                  Jennie Walls, R.N.C., M.S.N, F.N.C., Yoakley Hall, Rm. 209, 439-7143
                  Celesta Kirk, R.N., M.S.N., F.N.P., Yoakley Hall, Rm. 110, 439-7154
                  Bonnie Godfrey, M.S.N., J.D., Lamb Hall, Rm. 390, 439-

                  [Family/Community department telephone number is 439-4484]

PLACEMENT: Senior Level

CREDIT: 5 Semester Hours

PRE-COREQUISITE: FCNU 4210

CATALOG DESCRIPTION:
Opportunity for the student to utilize the nursing process with clients in the community
setting. Includes study of community clients using assessment and planning skills to
enhance achievement of optimum level of wellness. Concepts of epidemiology, community
assessment, program planning, community networks, and community diagnoses are
discussed.

COURSE OVERVIEW:
This course focuses on the care of individuals, families and groups in home and community
settings by applying the nursing process, knowledge and abilities from previous courses.
Emphasis is placed on providing population-focused care, culturally relevant care, and on
the crisis theory goals of health promotion and disease prevention. Experiences are
planned to promote continued development of nursing competencies and their application
to community health nursing. Students will have opportunities to experience the nurses'
roles of case finder, care provider, service coordinator, collaborator, consultant, advocate,
health program planner and health educator.

STUDENT PROCEDURES FOR SPECIAL SERVICES:
Students who have special needs as a result of a disability should contact the Director for
Disabled Students Services, D.P. Culp University Center, phone 929-4841.

TEXTBOOKS:

Stanhope, M., & Lancaster, J. (1996). *Community health nursing: Process and practice for
promoting health*, 4th ed. St. Louis: Mosby. (required)

Lorig, K. (1996). *Patient education: A practical approach*, 2nd ed. Thousand Oaks: Sage. (recommended)

COURSE OUTCOMES:
At the conclusion of the course the student will be able to:

1. Implement strategies designed to promote the health of individuals and families within the context of community as client, using nursing process, critical thinking/diagnostic reasoning skills, and therapeutic communication.

2. Implement effective strategies to promote the health of communities or selected populations at risk, using nursing process, critical thinking/diagnostic reasoning skills, and therapeutic communication.

3. Work in partnership with clients in the context of cultural and individual differences when planning, implementing, and evaluating community health nursing care.

4. Collaborate with other professionals when providing community health nursing care.

5. Use pertinent community resources that are consistent with clients' health care needs.

6. Incorporate research findings into specific plans of care.

7. Implement legal, ethical and professional standards of practice in providing nursing care.

LEARNING STRATEGIES:

1. Engage in clinical practice with individuals and families in primary care and community health settings 6 hours per week and complete the Clinical/Agency Experience Forms weekly.

2. Critique, in writing, one community health agency for nature of services, role of provider, strengths and weaknesses of services.

3. Observe and assist the public health nurse (PHN) or community health nurse (CHN) in their activities in various agencies. Rotations will be scheduled by the instructors.

4. Participate in scheduled faculty-student conferences to promote collaborative peer learning.

5. Develop a family care plan based on a family assessment and family diagnoses, using a videotaped interview.

6. Collaborate with peers and members of a designated aggregate group at risk, for approximately 6 hours weekly, to plan, implement and evaluate programs to meet identified health needs of the at-risk group.

7.   Write a comprehensive paper about the aggregate project using the stated specific guidelines to describe the collaborative assessment and implementation process, including clinical decisions, rationale for priorities and the plan of evaluation.

EVALUATION METHODS:

		Due Date
Medication examination	P/F	9-11-96
Evaluation of clinical practice competencies related to individuals, families.	P/F	
Clinic critique	20%	9-16-96
Family Care Plan	20%	10-28-96
Aggregate Project	60%	
Draft Part I		9-23-96
Final Part I		10-7-96
Part II		11-4-96
Total	100%	

(See specific guidelines for each assignment)

The grading scale used to determine the practicum grade is: A=100-92%   B=91-83%   C=82-75%

Notes:

A passing score must be obtained on the medication exam by 9/11/96. One retake of the examination will be allowed. A student must have satisfactory ratings from each clinic and community-based preceptor <u>and</u> from their clinical instructor in order to pass the course.

Up to 15 points may be deducted for any written assignment that does not comply with standard use of English language, format, spelling, sentence and paragraph structure, or content relevant to the topic. Plagiarized texts of others may results in failure of the course.
Five points will be deducted each day for assignments turned in past the due date.

An <u>unexcused absence</u> (such as an absence without prior notification to appropriate persons, or unmet health requirements) will result in a lowering of the final grade by one letter grade. Two unexcused absences will result in failure of the course.

GENERAL COURSE POLICIES: Throughout the community health nursing practicum, the student is expected to:

1. Provide own transportation to and from the clinical sites.

2. Report any foreseen absence to both the faculty preceptor and the agency contact person at the earliest feasible time in order to reschedule your responsibilities. Excused clinical absences will be made up at the faculty preceptor's discretion.

3. Take the scheduled assessment test offered by the Student Resources Center as partial fulfillment of the course. Time required for the examination can be counted as practicum time (see Student Handbook, "NCLEX Exam"). This applies only to generic baccalaureate students.

4. Comply with designated protocols about your specific rotation, including what to wear, the scheduled time, and your responsibilities. Read this information in the Agency Description Notebook <u>before</u> your assigned clinical day. A notebook will be available from each clinical instructor (or at the clinical site) and C. Macnee's (Room 212 - Yoakley) door, and on reserve at Sherrod Library. <u>Prepare for clinical by reviewing material as indicated.</u>

5. Give a Clinic Preceptor Evaluation Form along with a stamped envelope which is addressed to the clinical faculty to each agency preceptor to complete. The preceptor will complete this form after you leave and will mail it to your instructor. (Students are responsible for making copies of this form and for providing the stamped and addressed envelopes.)

6. Schedule community and student group meetings so they do not conflict with other courses.

7. Make a concerted effort to visit families at home and communicate to your instructor difficulty in finding families at home within a reasonable time period in the clinical day.

8. In the event of inclement weather like snow or ice, students must use their own prudent judgement about classroom attendance. Contact your instructor and agency contact person if you can not drive safely to clinical during inclement weather. Clinical absences will be made up at a later date in collaboration with your instructor.

9. Develop contingency plans with aggregate groups in the event of inclement weather.

FCNU 4211

Guidelines for the Clinic Critique

Clinic Critique (20% of total 4211 grade)

Each student will analyze one clinic or community-based experience. The purpose of the clinic critique is to examine critically (use your critical thinking skills!) how the CHN/PHN provides population-focused care within the context of a clinic or community-based setting. Use your observation and critical thinking skills for this assignment. The instructor is interested in what you think about the clinic -- in your ability to analyze the strengths and weaknesses of the clinic in terms of providing population-focused care.

Write the critique in narrative APA format; it must be typed and double spaced. The critique should be concise yet pithy. Points will be deducted if a critique exceeds 5 pages including cover page. The critique is due September 16, 1996.

A. Describe the clinic or community-based nursing setting in terms of: (20 points)

  – Purpose of clinic
  – Target Population (the group of people the clinic is meant to benefit). Describe what characteristics this population shares
  – Clinic services and strategies for primary, secondary, and/or tertiary levels of prevention (give specific examples of services provided for each level of prevention)

B. Critique the clinic or community-based nursing setting by exploring the following: (80 points; 20 points each)

  – Strengths of the clinic
  – Barriers/dilemmas associated with providing population-focused care for clinic staff
  – Barriers/dilemmas faced by members of the target population (associated with receiving services)
  – Suggestions for improving the clinic's effectiveness in providing population-focused care (constructive, realistic suggestions given the realities of the clinic or community-based setting.)

Give specific examples for all sections requested in Part B

Student Comments

Portions of some students' Fall '95 reflection papers are highlighted below. Comments culled from student responses to the question: "Has this course created any changes in your life, your goals, or your values?"

Thanks for the terrific class -- and for putting me in touch with the helping side of myself again!

First [sic] the first time in my life, I was actually disappointed because a class wasn't meeting. I liked the class, I loved the teacher, and I changed bunches -- that should be enough.

I also have become aware that one person can make a difference even if only a little at a time. I really enjoyed the homeless breakfast I attended and plan to try to start a similar program at my church because of this experience.

This class has taught me how truly enjoyable volunteer work can be. I always wondered why people would want to work and not be paid for it, but since I've been volunteering at NET (North East Tennessee Academy) I have really enjoyed and I don't think about the fact that I'm not paid for it because I don't think of it as a job. I plan to continue volunteering there after this class is finished because I see these boys as friends, not as just delinquents and I thouroughly (sic) enjoy the volunteer work.

By taking this class I have come to realize my true feelings regarding such issues as race relations, sexual orientations, and the unique differences of individuals. I have never had a class that has discussed these topics. I finally realized how I feel because I verbally discussed it. Once it came out of my lips, in my own words, it brought my true feelings to the surface.

I have never experienced a class that I felt that I truly could say anything (almost) that I believe in. My eyes have been opened to many problems in our "small" town. I think most of all I enjoyed hearing the way other classmates feel about different issues, especially race. (Note: The student is African-American.)

I never have been angry about welfare and other ways that people receive (sic) money, but I am open minded and have considered other ideas. The change that has occured (sic) in me is even a closer understanding than I had before.

I enjoyed this class and getting close to other fellow students has helped me grown personally and enhance my ability to become a team member.

I have really gotten to know the children that I am tutoring at Towne Acres a lot (sic). They look forward to my coming and talking to them.

This course is the most significant course on ETSU's campus! It's allowed me to explore career ideas and make a career decision.

Feeding the homeless had really opened my eyes. I was amazed at the fact that homeless trully (sic) exists ... I especially enjoyed the Thank You's from the homeless individuals; The impact of that situation is a experience of a lifetime.

I have thoroughly enjoyed this class. It has made me open to other views and ideas. I would say that I was homophobic when I came into this class, but I feel that I have started to overcome that. Though it is not a lifestyle that I condone or believe in I can learn to deal with it. Race issues is another thing that I have learned to accept better.

This class has helped me socially, mentally and has been a tremendous help with me dealing with the public again.

I have had a major life change. I've been sober since 9/25. The positive feed back from my teacher on my second paper as I told in writing about my drinking problem. Thank you! I also feel I've been taught to be more assertive, freer to express my feelings and thoughts. I never had a role model or someone to look up to, but I think I found one. My teacher Mrs. Duncan. I would like to be more out going and assertive.

I think this has been a wonderful class. I've learned that I can make a difference in my community and that my voice counts. I have also learnt (sic) that a class can be fun and so can learning.

This class has made me much more aware of how I can participate in society. It is not as hard as it may seem. If everyone would take just a small step as we have in this class, it would create a huge impact on our society as a whole.

Having only been in this class for the past six weeks, I can already see the effect it has had and will have on my life. It has taught me the importance of working for your community and the positive effect just one person can have. Not only this, but I'm learning an immense amount from my peers in the class. Ms. Duncan has created an open and comfortable environment for us to exchange ideas, beliefs, feelings, and things we've learned from our placements. It only takes one visit to this class to see the bond between the students with each other and with the teacher. Through this bond, I've been able to learn so much about things such as prejudices, the importance of open communication, being informed about the world, and how to handle certain people and/or situations. This is the first class that truly integrates real-life experience with the classroom. The things I'm learning from this class are invaluable.

Materials From Service-Learning Courses on Homelessness and Rural Nursing

by Suzanne MacAvoy, the Rev. Paul E. Carrier, and Elizabeth Gardner

Contents

FP 125   Homelessness: Causes and Consequences

Faculty: Suzanne MacAvoy, RN, EdD
Rev. Paul E. Carrier, SJ, PhD
Elizabeth Gardner, PhD

Description:

Students will use theory, field experiences, reflection, and critical analysis to broaden and deepen their understanding of homelessness and homeless people. The causes and consequences of homelessness will be discussed from a variety of perspectives, with particular emphasis on ethics, social justice, and mental, physical, psychological, and spiritual health. We will discuss the effects of homelessness on individuals, families, and society, and examine both short-range and long-range interventions and solutions.

Each week there will be three hours of seminar, in which students are expected to participate actively, and three hours of field placements outside of class periods which are required as part of the homework. During seminars, we will discuss readings and videotapes, hear a variety of guest speakers, share our experiences in field placements, and integrate them with theory through discussions, critical reflection papers, and other assignments. Field placements may include shelters, soup kitchens, child care centers, drop-in centers, and other settings. Students will do a project on homelessness and present the project in class.

Grading:

Participation (including discussion of required and supplemental readings, issues, experiences;
journal; insight cards) - 25%
Critical reflection papers (10) - 40%
Individual Final Project and Presentation - 25% + 10%

Required Texts:

Jencks, C. (1994). *The homeless.* Cambridge, MA: Harvard University Press.
Kozol, J. (1988). *Rachel and her children: Homeless families in America.* New York: Fawcett Columbine.
Smith, G.N. (1994). *Street journal: Finding God in the homeless.* Kansas City, MO: Sheed and Ward.
Wright, J.D. (1989). *Address unknown: The homeless in America.* New York: Aldine de Gruyter.
Baum, A. S. and Burnes, D. W. (1994). *A nation in denial.* San Francisco: Westview Press.

Class Schedule:

Unit I   What is homelessness? (3 classes)
Unit II   Who are the homeless? (3 classes)
Unit III   Origins of homelessness - Economics, Mental Illness, Substance Abuse, Social Networks (4
classes)
Unit IV   Ideological underpinnings - Ethics, spirituality, faith, justice (4 classes)
Unit V   Impact of homelessness on the homeless - Women and Children, Health, Coping (3 classes)
Unit VI   Interventions (4 classes)
Student project presentations (4 classes)

-2-

Field Experiences:

Field experiences will take place in one of the following sites:
 Prospect House, Bridgeport
 Pacific House, Stamford
 St. Luke's Community Services, Stamford
 Thomas Merton House, Bridgeport
 Gillespie House, Westport
 Alpha Home, Bridgeport
 Operation Hope, Fairfield

Faculty will meet with you during the first week of class to discuss your objectives, preferences, and skills and help you select the field placement best suited to you. You will spend approximately 3 hours each week at your site. The time and the activities will vary depending upon your schedule and that of the site.

Assignments:

1. Individual Final Project:

Each student will do a project on homelessness that relates to the course content and that incorporates learning from field experiences. Faculty will serve as advisors in project development and implementation. Quality of literature support and exposition will be included in the evaluation of the project.
 The focus or topic may be from the following list or an idea of your own. You may find it helpful to select a topic related to your site or the population they serve. The topic should be discussed with and approved by one of the faculty.
 A paper or written report will be prepared for the project. Presentation of the projects will be scheduled towards the end of the semester.

Topic/Focus:
 (a) Monitor the media (newspapers, news magazines, TV, etc.) over the course of the semester. Identify and critically analyze issues, concerns, trends, etc. as they emerge over the semester. Relate what you are reading/seeing/hearing in the media to what you are learning in class and experiencing in your field experiences. Develop a position and/or action plan regarding issues.
 (b) Explore an issue, concern, etc related to homelessness in a particular community, including causes, problems, ramifications, resources, solutions, etc. This may involve interviewing and data collection from social service personnel, volunteers, homeless persons, and/or others. Develop a position and/or action plan regarding the issue.
 (c) Walk in another's shoes by spending long periods of time with one or two homeless people, getting to know them and experiencing what they experience as they live without a home, seek support from social agencies, travel from place to place without a base, deal with maintaining dignity and self esteem, etc. Write of your responses to your vicarious and first-hand experiences, including coping strategies and other helping or hindering forces you encounter and/or observe.
 (d) Conduct a series of seminars or classes or develop a video program for others, to heighten their awareness about homelessness in its multiple dimensions. The target audience may be another student population - preschool, school age, adolescent, peer, or an adult group. The setting may be a school system, youth group, church group, senior group, or a community organization.
 (e) Interview people who are in a position to influence services for, or public opinion of, the homeless, e.g., mayor/selectpersons, Attorney General, state and city legislators, police, editors, directors

of agencies, etc. Compare and contrast their perceptions, policies, and perspectives with what you are learning in class, through readings, and in field experiences.

(f) Come up with an idea of your own.

2. Journal:

What is a journal? It's about you. The journal reflects the content of those moments in time that have a special meaning for you; experiences from which you draw understanding about yourself and your world.

The one person you need to get to know very well in this world is you. The journal can be an excellent teacher. Putting into words your experiences, thoughts, and feelings can cause you to reflect more on your life. Writing about yourself is one way to grow in knowing yourself, to become aware of your learning, and to understand why you do the things you do.

What is important is to share ideas, work out your thoughts and create. The journal is more than a point by point description of activities, it is also how you think and feel about what you are doing.

1. Use a special notebook.

2. Be specific. The journal will be used in supervision meetings.

3. Be complete; describe; reflect.

3. Weekly Critical Reflection Paper:

This is a capsule critical essay written as a response to and analysis of the readings, discussions, field experiences. The purpose of this essay is to allow you to articulate your understanding of a particular topic or theme.

Focus -- a couple of key points; agree, disagree, elaborate, refer to readings to make connections.

Begin with a brief introduction, say what you are planning to do in your paper. Do it, follow an outline of your ideas. Don't assume anything, not even the intelligence of your readers. Wrap it up; bring it to closure. Did you say what you wanted to say?

2-3 pages, double spaced

Ns 362
Rural Nursing in Appalachia

Faculty: Suzanne MacAvoy, RN, EdD

Description: This course focuses on rural nursing in Appalachia, in particular the culture and mores of the area, the impact of rural poverty on health, and the health problems and nursing diagnoses common in people of the eastern Kentucky region of Appalachia.

Objectives:
1. Describe the culture of the people of eastern KY and Appalachia.
2. Describe various effects of rural poverty and cultural values on health.
3. Discuss common health problems and nursing diagnoses of people living in eastern KY.
4. Describe the role of the nurse in rural health.

Class Content:
I   Culture and mores of Appalachia: Historical, geographical, political
II Rural poverty
       Economic implications
       Access to health care
       Role of nurse in rural health
       Frontier Nursing Service
III Common health care needs
       Wound healing, skin ulcers
       Pneumoconiosis
       Undernutrition, Obesity
IV Nursing diagnoses and interventions
       Impaired skin/tissue integrity
       Activity intolerance
       Altered health/home maintenance
       Ineffective airway clearance/breathing pattern
       Over/undernutrition
       Compliance/non-compliance
       Management of therapeutic regimen

Assignments:
1. Book/video report
2. Critical reflection paper
   a. Select one health care problem prevalent in Appalachia. (You are not restricted to the ones discussed in class - other common problems are abuse, alcoholism, hyperlipidemia, diabetes, lung cancer, breast cancer, dental caries, anxiety, depression, prenatal care, low birth weight, teen suicide, health promotion, smoking, drug use, or others you may encounter through your reading.)
   b. Discuss nursing care needed by clients with this health problem.
   c. Describe interrelationships of culture and poverty with this health problem and the impact of these on the clients ability to improve their health status. Describe how characteristics and strengths can be used to improve health.
   d. Include current references and current research.
   e. If also enrolled in Ns 364, select one nursing care area (related to the health care problem selected above) that was a challenge or which required special consideration with one of your patients, e.g., health teaching, self care, environmental factors, compliance, etc. Also include clinical examples to illustrate your points.

Ns 364
Clinical Practice in Appalachia

Faculty: Suzanne MacAvoy, RN, EdD

Description:

This clinical course is taken concurrently with Ns 362 Rural Nursing in Appalachia. Students will spend one week in Appalachia (spring break) working with public health nurses as they care for residents in the community. Enrollment is limited and by permission of the faculty.

Objectives:

1.   Relate knowledge of rural health, Appalachia and selected medical and nursing diagnoses, to patient care.
2.   Collaborate with public health nurses in St. Claire's Home Care Center in caring for clients.

Clinical experiences:

Students will spend one week in Morehead, Kentucky working with the public health nurses in Home Care at St. Claire's Medical Center. You will have an opportunity to visit the Outreach Clinics located in the rural counties surrounding Morehead. Conferences will include discussion and reflection on the experiences encountered in clinical practice, the interaction of poverty and culture on health status, and application of related theory to nursing care.

Assignments:

1.   <u>Journal:</u>
Keeping a journal gives you an opportunity to reflect upon those experiences which have special meaning for you, from which you draw understanding about yourself and your world. Putting into words your experiences, thoughts, and feelings can cause you to reflect more on your life. Writing about yourself is one way to grow in knowing yourself, to become aware of your learning, and to understand why you do the things you do.

What is important is to share ideas, work out your thoughts, and create. The journal is more than a point by point description of activities. It is also how you think and feel about what you are doing. Be specific. You will use your journal in your critical reflection paper.

2.   <u>Case study presentation:</u>
Each student will do a written case study and in-class presentation of the case study, at the end of the semester. Include personal, social and health history, discussion of medical and nursing diagnoses and care. Include socioeconomic and/or cultural factors that impacted on the health or care of the client.

3.   <u>Critical reflection paper:</u>
When you do your critical reflection paper for Ns 362,
        (a) select a health care problem you encountered while in Appalachia,
        (b) include clinical examples to illustrate points, and
        (c) include reflections from your journal.

Set 4

Materials From Service-Learning Practica in Nursing Service Administration

by Linda Workman, L. Sue Davis, and Darlene A. Anderson

Contents

University of Cincinnati
College of Nursing and Health

Faculty: L. Sue Davis, RN, PhD

Community Health Nursing Practica
Service-Learning Activities

Course Overviews and Objectives

Three Community Health Nursing practica courses offer graduate students opportunities to develop skills in needs assessment, program planning, program implementation and outcomes evaluation. Through these courses students integrate didactic learning with the realities of providing primary, secondary, and tertiary care to community-based populations. Objectives for each course are patterned on a planning, implementation, and evaluation process that also patterns the didactic courses. Courses differ only in the population level need (primary, secondary, tertiary) or the management need. Objectives are sufficiently abstract to allow for negotiation of a project that meets both student learning needs and agency service needs. In the contracting process, students are expected to identify their learning needs and clearly identify the "product" to be offered to the agency.

Practicum in Primary Prevention with Communities

The first practicum, Primary Prevention (29-566-844) focuses on concepts and principles of health promotion, disease prevention, and risk reduction. The purpose is to enhance the well-being of a targeted population. Schools, parishes, nursing clinics, wellness centers, senior centers, primary care sites, employment settings, radio and television stations are frequently used as sites. Experiences may be either rural or urban. Interdisciplinary projects with masters students in environmental health, health education, and women's studies are encouraged.

Course Objectives:
1. Analyze assessment data acquired from a target population for the purpose of identifying a health promotion or a risk reduction need.
2. Identify priorities for program implementation by establishing criteria for prioritizing health promotion needs or risks of the identified population.
3. Develop primary nursing intervention plans specific to identified priorities.
4. Implement the plan for primary prevention.
5. Evaluate actual outcomes of the health promotion/risk reduction interventions in terms of the desired outcomes.

Practicum in Secondary and Tertiary Prevention with Communities

The second practicum, Secondary and Tertiary Prevention (29-566-850) focuses on populations experiencing acute or chronic health needs. Using crisis, family, and developmental theories, along with case management concepts, students design, implement and/or evaluate interventions aimed at early detection, intervention and referral, disability limitation, and assistance with recovery and rehabilitation. An interdisciplinary approach is emphasized and projects may be jointly undertaken with masters students in environmental health, health policy, or social work.

Course Objectives:
1. Identify sources of data for factors impacting secondary and tertiary health needs and analyze the limitations of the data.
2. Gather and analyze assessment data from an at risk target population.

1

3.   Identify priorities for intervention by establishing criteria for prioritizing health needs of the population.
4.   Develop and implement a nursing protocol for the management of a selected population.
5.   Evaluate actual outcomes in terms of the predicted outcomes.
6.   Forecast the benefits of the protocol to the health of the targeted population in relation to socio-cultural, psychological, physical, and economical forces within the environment.

<u>Practicum in Leadership, Structure & Politics in Community Health Agencies</u>

The third practicum, Leadership, Structure and Politics (29-566-848) focuses on application of management concepts and the role of the health service manager in program planning, implementation and evaluation. An interdisciplinary approach is emphasized and projects may be jointly undertaken with masters students in health service administration.

Course Objectives:
1.   Analyze assessment data acquired from a nursing management perspective for the purpose of identifying health service management needs.
2.   Analyze assessment data and establish criteria for prioritizing health service management needs.
3.   Identify potential barriers and constraints to successful implementation of the management project.
4.   Develop management/program plans specific to identified priorities.
5.   Develop evaluation plan consistent with management/program goals and objectives.
6.   Implement identified plan.
7.   Provide agency with written and verbal management/project reports at completion of contracted project.

In each practicum, students are in the position of representing the College of Nursing and Health. Professional conduct and appearance are expected at all times. Students are reminded that the host institution is entitled to complete confidentiality, and confidentiality statements are signed when proprietary information is accessed. No proper names of individuals or organizations are used on any written work, nor is discussion of internal organizational matters outside of the educational context allowed.

Operationalization of the Practica and Related Service Learning Activities

Practica courses are offered winter and spring quarter, allowing time in the fall to solicit projects from community-based agencies. Although this is done formally through written communication, agencies often call to request students for special projects. The process of solicitation allows for development of a "bank" of service projects which can be screened for appropriateness, scope, and area of learning. Students may select from available projects or they may choose to develop a project on their own. Agencies are asked to financially support the material costs of the project and provide the student with recognition of effort. All three practica may be completed in one agency or in three different agencies, depending on the student's learning goals. Larger projects may be undertaken by a group of students, thereby offering the opportunity to enhance group process skills.

Because of the interdisciplinary nature of the program of study, academic contacts are maintained with other University departments, such as Health Education, Social Work, Environmental Health, and Health Services Administration. Projects are often enhanced by including students from other disciplines. This reduces faculty effort directed toward course project development, but increases effort in planning, coordination, and supervision of Service-Learning projects.

The student(s), supervising professor, and agency representatives meet to discuss the service project. This meeting allows service provider and student the opportunity to reach mutual goals and expectations. The professor most

2

often functions as an "interpreter" between the educational and service cultures, and assists both domains to set reasonable objectives and time frames. The student(s) are then expected to develop a project plan, which is presented at a second meeting with the service agency and professor. Expectations are finalized and a contract signed by students, professor, and agency preceptor.

Projects are supervised through meetings with students every two weeks in which implementation plans are reviewed against accomplished milestones. One page progress reports, in the form of a memo, are submitted to the preceptor. Students complete one formative and one summative self-evaluation. They evaluate the agency in the areas of learning climate, availability of resources, and availability of preceptor. Preceptors evaluate the project in relation to appropriateness of student interaction, timeliness of reports, and usefulness of finished project to the institution.

Project reports consist of (a) defined goals, (b) measurable outcome parameters, (c) review of the literature and data sources, (d) project and evaluation plan, (e) presentation of findings and data analysis, (f) implications and recommendations, (g) appendices - interventions, additional data, etc. Examples of Service-learning projects are listed below:

1.   An empowerment project for assisting a community center develop and implement a health promotion program for participants.

2.   Data collection and analysis for a subcommittee of a large community group conducting a community health status assessment.

3.   Development and implementation of a wellness program for older adults with alcoholism.

4.   Conducting a community analysis of emergency room use for a managed care group.

5.   Developing, implementing, and evaluating a documentation system for parish nursing.

6.   Identifying populations at-risk in a major Medicaid HMO and developing intervention strategies for those populations.

7.   Developing an evaluation plan for a case management model for a working population.

8.   Conducting a health needs assessment, and developing and integrating an arthritis self-care program into a wellness center for older adults.

3

University of Cincinnati
College of Nursing and Health

Faculty: Linda L. Workman, RN, PhD
Darlene A. Anderson, RN, DNSc

Nursing Services Administrative Practica
Service-Learning Activities

Course Overviews and Objectives

The three administrative practica in the graduate program provide opportunities for students to develop managerial skills and to integrate theory with the realities of clinical practice. In addition, the intensive working relationship with the preceptor provides a rich opportunity for role development. The course objectives for the practica are sufficiently broad, to be interpreted in terms of students' educational needs, resources, and interests, and to be met in a wide variety of clinical contacts. Each practica has a distinct focus with the second practicum building upon the first, and the third practicum building upon the second. For each practicum, students negotiate a relevant learning contract with the graduate faculty supervisor and the administrative preceptor.

The **first practicum (29-595-837)** has a comprehensive focus on analyzing the structural, functional, and human resource system of a health services organization. Skill development specific to human resources management function is elaborated on, including methods/ techniques used for acquiring, developing, evaluating, and compensating human resources. In addition, alternative leadership styles and strategies are examined and critiqued as students work on their own role development.

Course Objectives:

1. Evaluate the nursing service departmental structure relative to implementation of the philosophy and goals.
2. Evaluate standards of care and patient outcomes in relation to departmental structure and function and external criteria, e.g., JCAHO, Medicaid, Medicare, etc.
3. Analyze the human resource management and labor relation practices within the nursing department and organization.
4. Apply management concepts in the identification and completion of relevant project(s) identified and approved by their faculty preceptor.

The **second practicum (29-595-838)** is focused on analyzing the role of the departmental manager and/or selective agency executives in the management of financial resources. Skill development specific to developing and implementing the annual operational budget for a department and/or agency is elaborated on, including methods for calculating revenues and expenses, maintaining financial control, and evaluating performance outcomes. In addition, strategies for improving productivity and service quality are explored.

Course Objectives:

1. Analyze fiscal parameters in relation to established quality and productivity indicators for a specific unit and/or department.
2. Contrast patient care delivery system/model used within the nursing department/unit with new and/or evolving professional practice models.
3. Evaluate the methods used in determining and allocating human resources in relation to patient care delivery and the decision support systems.

1

4.   Evaluate the philosophy and practices of the nursing department/units specific to recruitment and retention, e.g., staff development, career ladder, etc.
5.   Evaluate congruence of quality assurance/improvement programs within the department of nursing in relation to standards of nursing practice, patient care standards, and accreditation requirements.
6.   Apply management concepts in the identification and completion of relevant project(s) identified and approved by their faculty preceptor.

The **third practicum (29-595-839)** is focused on analyzing the role of departmental manager and/or selective agency executives in the strategic management function. Skill development specific to developing and implementing the strategic business plan of a health services organization is elaborated on, including the various methods/techniques used for assessing an organization's competitive position, informing strategic choices, and managing cultural change necessary for the successful implementation of the chosen strategy. Emphasis is placed on demonstrating the use of strategic concepts and models through the design and completion of an administrative project approved by the preceptor and faculty supervisor.

Course Objectives:

1.   Analyze the impact of organizational structure and institutional policies on the role of the nurse administrator.
2.   Evaluate nursing service administration role in strategic management.
3.   Differentiate nursing care delivery from health care delivery for purposes of strategic planning.
4.   Analyze external factors (environmental, competition, socio-cultural, political, regulatory and/or labor relations, financial, etc.) which affect administrative decisions related to nursing and health care delivery.
5.   Identify strategies which facilitate maintenance and progressive practices within the nursing department.
6.   Identify strategies which facilitate maintenance and progressive practices between nursing service and other departments and/or within the corporate structure.
7.   Utilize concepts of advance practice developed through research and practice in formulating decisions.
8.   Demonstrate use of administrative strategies through the design and implementation of a nursing project identified with and approved by faculty and preceptor.

In all practica, students are in the position of representing both the College of Nursing and Health, and on occasion, the administrative preceptor in the host institution. Professional conduct and appearance are expected at all times. In addition, students are reminded that the host institution is entitled to complete confidentiality. No proper names of individuals or organizations are used on any written work nor is discussion of internal organizational matters outside of the education context allowed.

Operationalization of the Practica and Related Service-Learning Activities

The NSA Practica are arranged to facilitate Service-learning opportunities for students. These are accomplished through a number of activities. First, the courses have been organized so that experiences flow from basic understanding of the Nursing/Patient Care Department within an organization to a complex analysis of issues and processes operationally defined within and external to the department and/or organization. Second, continuity of learning is facilitated by having the students assigned to the same institution and nursing service administrator/preceptor for the three Practica experiences. Third, student learning is targeted at an organizational level above the position they currently hold and/or left, prior to returning to school full time. Fourth, student placement is arranged in an organization other than their current place of employment.

2

The placement of the students is based on an evaluation of the individual student's learning needs. This evaluation is completed through a joint meeting of the student and faculty member. Factors considered in the evaluation include: (a) the student's current level of knowledge and/or job responsibilities, (b) past work experiences, (c) the student's desires for future employment, and (d) the availability of nursing administrative preceptors in areas of the student's interests. Once the goals for learning have been defined, the student is provided the names of potential preceptors and their places of employment. The student is instructed to arrange a meeting with these potential preceptors to discuss learning goals and opportunities within the practice setting. This meeting also provides both the student and the preceptor a chance to evaluate one another for "fit." Once the preceptor and placement have been decided upon, the student is expected to develop goals for the three practica experiences. Next, a meeting is arranged between the student, nursing administrative preceptor, and the faculty member. In this meeting the expectations for all parties are defined and a contract for the experience is signed.

Although the syllabi have clearly defined objectives for each experience, the student and preceptor are allowed flexibility to adjust outcomes across the three practica. This is done to meet the learning needs available within the department and/or organization based on a given quarter, e.g., budget development may not occur in Fall quarter so the student would be allowed to wait until Winter or Spring quarter to meet that objective. In addition, since all learning needs may not have been identified or were not available at the time of the initial contract, ongoing adjustments may be made in the learning contract. These changes are negotiated by the student with their preceptor and communicated and approved by faculty. In addition, each student is expected to complete at least one major project for their preceptor and/or within the organization per experience. The project(s) have taken numerous forms. On occasion the student will be involved in a major departmental or organizational undertaking, such as, movement to patient focused care, creation of a shared governance model, etc. In these experiences the student's involvement and role specific to the project would be continuous with a more advanced/in depth project occurring with each experience. In other situations the student may be asked to do single and/or multiple projects per experience. The number of learning expectations are based on the knowledge, ability and interest of the student, and support availability for each project.

Examples of students' projects are listed below:

1.   Quality Assessment Study: Patient call lights for 5 CD & 4AB/Emmanuel Unit.

2.   Evaluation of baseline FTE (FT and PT) requirements per clinical unit complete with stated assumptions and computer assisted program for ongoing evaluation.

3.   A comparison of the knowledge acquisition in adult female clients following individual or videotape instruction about colposcopy in an outpatient setting.

4.   Evaluation of a healthcare technician program including: (a) previous work experience, (b) training and orientation effectiveness and costs for currently employed healthcare technicians recruited - internal and external, (c) evaluation of retention, e.g., turnover and cost, and (d) evaluation of nurse preceptor effectiveness and satisfaction specific to the training of healthcare technician within a given organization.

5.   Comparison of the nurse manager's actual work, using the Nursing Work Survey Instrument, and expected work as defined by the nurse manager job description.

These and other projects were completed by students working with their preceptors. They consisted of (a) clearly defined purpose and/or problem statement, (b) defined outcome parameters for the projects, (c) review of the relevant literature, (d) data analysis, and (e) cost analysis, if appropriate. Each of the projects also resulted in a formalized written document and, in many cases, verbal presentations.

3

The faculty member assigned to each student, although not on site, is involved throughout the experience. This involvement consists of at least three on site visits per quarter, review of the student's weekly log, verbal reports from the student and/or nursing administrative preceptor, review of completed student project(s) and/or presentations, and through course evaluations submitted by both the student and preceptor. These activities allow the faculty to continuously assess the student's progress and to help in identifying other learning experiences that would enhance the student's learning.

4

University of Cincinnati
College of Nursing and Health

Faculty: Linda L. Workman, RN, PhD
Darlene A. Anderson, RN, DNSc
Linda Sue Davis, RN, PhD

Master's Thesis/Projects
Service-Learning Activities

This experience as designed is a capstone experience. The learning opportunity is therefore directed at a research question and/or project which will allow the student to apply the knowledge gained throughout their program of study. According to the guidelines developed within the College of Nursing and Health, thesis and project experience have been defined as the same process except that the latter involves two or three students working together on the same project.

Use of the project experience has provided some interesting learning experiences for students and faculty and has facilitated objective analysis and plan development for nursing/patient care services administrators within the community. That is, faculty working with groups of students have taken on agency projects as a focus of analysis and/or ongoing study. For the most part these projects have focused on evaluation research methods. The projects usually have an institutional or departmental focus, thus allowing for six to eight students to be involved in a given project/study. The projects as developed are coordinated by the faculty with subsets of the projects being assigned to groups of two to three students. This allows faculty to mentor students through the capstone experience and provides students with a readily available project for completion of their course requirement. In addition, it facilitates the students' ability to (a) work in groups, (b) understand and manage project subsets, (c) develop a formal document and presentation, and (d) understand the magnitude of a larger aggregate study and its use by a department/agency in addressing an issue and/or making change. It further facilitates both the student and the department/agency in meeting their desired outcomes.

Some examples of graduate projects conducted by students and faculty within the nursing service administration major are listed below.

1. Comparison of budgeted to actual nursing staff positions allocated per unit and their distribution across shifts for the purpose of staffing.

2. Development of a work survey instrument for use in the measurement of nursing work. (This project involved 12 students (six groups of two students each) focusing on comprehensive literature and practice review and on pilot testing of an instrument to determine instrument reliability and validity.)

3. Analysis of work completed by nursing personnel in the inpatient units utilizing the Nursing Work Survey Instrument. (This project involved 10 students (five groups of two students each) and focused on analysis of two inpatient units per student group.)

4. Analysis of work completed by professional nurses, psychiatric social workers, nonprofessional staff, and nurse managers in a psychiatric emergency center utilizing the Nursing Work Survey Instrument. (This project involved two students.)

5. Analysis of work completed by professional nurses, technical staff, and nurse managers in a perioperative setting utilizing the Nursing Work Survey Instrument. (This project involved two students.)

1

6. Analysis of charted nursing interventions grouped by nursing intervention categories (NICs) compared to classified acuity indicators and defined functional care categories for patients on:

    A. Total Hip Replacement (DRG 209) clinical pathway. (This project involved three students.)

    B. Percutaneous Transluminal Coronary Angioplasty (DRG 112) clinical pathway. (This project involved three students.)

7. Comparison of nurse and patient satisfaction, physician and nurse collaboration, and quality of care on two inpatient units:

    A. A renal/transplant surgery unit and a general medical unit. (This project involved two students.)

    B. An infectious disease unit and a medical-surgical unit. (This project involved two students.)

    C. An oncology-general medicine unit and a neuroscience unit. (This project involved two students.)

    D. A general/orthopedic surgery unit and a gynecology/oncology surgery unit. (This project involved two students.)

It should also be noted that these and other learning opportunities have contributed to the graduation of 40 graduate students in the nursing service administration and community health nursing majors in the past five years. In addition, it has provided faculty an opportunity to continue to develop in their areas of specialty and to establish a line of inquiry that supports research interests and grant application.

2

Nursing and Service-Learning

by Gail Robinson

Community Partnerships

Barnett, Lynn. (1996). *Community Outreach in Associate Degree Nursing Programs*. Washington, DC: American Association of Community Colleges.
    Describes five community college associate's degree nursing programs that addressed community needs and demonstrated strong partnerships with local health-care providers; includes project summaries, success factors, challenges, and resources.

Carignan, Ann M. (1992). "Community College–Nursing Home Partnership: Impact on Nursing Care." *Geriatric Nursing* 13(3): 139-141.
    Reports on a survey of nursing home directors involved in a partnership project with six community colleges; details major areas of impact on professional and nonprofessional care giving.

Couto, Richard. (1982). *Streams of Idealism and Health Care Innovation*. New York, NY: Teachers College Press.
    Relates a set of activities by community members and college students directed toward achieving social change at the community level, combining service-learning for students and community mobilization around various issues.

Dean, Hannah, and Jan L. Lee. (1995). "Service and Education: Forging a Partnership." *Nursing Outlook* 43(3): 119-123.
    Proposes partnerships between nursing service and education to foster innovation and cooperation in practice, education, and research; describes the partnership between a Veterans Health Administration health facility and a university school of nursing and the process used to build the collaborative relationship.

Dolloph, Frances, et al. (February 1995). "Meeting the Needs of a Rural Community for Registered Nurses." Paper presented at the Annual Conference on Workforce Training of the League for Innovation in the Community College, San Diego, CA.
> Describes college-community collaboration established by a county commission charged with determining funding for a two-year rural nursing program.

Flick, Louise H., et al. (1994). "Building Community for Health: Lessons From a Seven-Year-Old Neighborhood/University Partnership." *Health Education Quarterly* 21(3): 369-380.
> Describes a graduate program for community health nurses; recounts conflicts between community groups that proved to be powerful catalysts and potential barriers to the use of Freire's concepts in community organizing.

Gauthier, Mary Anne, and Peggy Matteson. (1995). "The Role of Empowerment in Neighborhood-Based Nursing Education." *Journal of .Nursing Education* 34(8): 390-395.
> Explores the use of lifelong learning and creative and critical thinking to empower nursing students to provide appropriate care within a diverse population and evolving health-care system.

Hartley, Celia L., et al. (1992). *Community College–Nursing Home Partnership: Improving Care Through Education. Annual Reports, 1988-1992.* Seattle, WA: Shoreline Community College.
> Summarizes actions taken to foster communication, organize faculty development, and analyze curricula.

Kretzmann, John P., and John L. McKnight. (1993). *Building Communities From the Inside Out: A Path Toward Finding and Mobilizing a Community's Assets.* Chicago, IL: ACTA Publications.
> Summarizes successful, practical, and useful examples of community-building initiatives; describes connecting community needs and assets through local citizens associations, community groups, government, business, philanthropic organizations, cultural organizations, and educational and religious institutions.

Tagliareni, M. Elaine, et al. (1991). "Participatory Clinical Education: Reconceptualizing the Clinical Learning Environment." *Nursing and Health Care* 12(5): 248-250, 261-263.
> Describes the outcomes of the Community College–Nursing Home Partnership project in different areas.

Zungolo, Eileen. (1994). "Interdisciplinary Education in Primary Care: The Challenge." *Nursing and Health Care* 15(6): 288-292.
> Depicts an interdisciplinary health-care project that places nursing students and medical students in neighborhood health centers for clinical experiences for primary care; portrays students engaging in interdisciplinary seminars, working together with patients and families, and planning projects.

Curriculum Development

American Medical Student Association/Foundation. (1995). *National Health Service Corps Educational Program for Clinical and Community Issues in Primary Care*. Reston, VA: American Medical Student Association/Foundation.
> Provides a series of educational materials and activities designed to interest health-professions students and practicing clinicians in providing primary-care services to medically underserved communities; helps current and future providers understand contemporary practice settings, social conditions, and disease patterns through experiential learning and problem solving.

Eraut, Michael, et al. (April 1996). "Mediating Scientific Knowledge Into Health Care Practice: Evidence From Pre-Registration Programmes in Nursing and Midwifery Education, and Recommendations for Future Curriculum Design." Paper presented at the annual meeting of the American Educational Research Association, New York, NY.
> Uses case studies to investigate the ways in which theoretical knowledge is taught and linked to professional health-care practice in a variety of curricula in educational settings and the ways in which the use of theory is introduced in service settings.

Jackson, Katherine, ed. (1994). *Redesigning Curricula: Models of Service Learning Syllabi*. Providence, RI: Campus Compact.
> Includes adaptable model syllabi from several disciplines at different types of institutions.

Kuennen, Jackie, and Vicki A. Moss. (1995). "Community Program Planning: A Clinical Outcome." *Journal of Nursing Education* 34(8): 387-389.
Relates the design of a community health project to help nursing students develop critical-thinking skills.

Larson, June. (1992). "The Healing Web: A Transformative Model for Nursing." *Nursing and Health Care* 13(5): 246-252.
Describes the Healing Web project, the goal of which is to create a values-based curriculum that could generate the support of nursing educators and nursing leaders.

Middlemiss, Mary Ann, and Jocelyne Van Neste Kenny. (1994). "Curriculum Revolution: Reflective Minds and Empowering Relationships." *Nursing and Health Care* 15(7): 350-353.
Examines the shift in curricular focus in nursing education, from objectives, outcomes, and evaluation to reflection, intuition, and praxis; depicts active learning as emphasizing constructing new knowledge and meaning, empowering students to take charge of their experience.

Noble, Mary Anne, et al. (1996). "Education for the Nurse of Tomorrow: A Community-Focused Curriculum." *Nursing and Health Care: Perspectives on Community* 17(2): 66-71.
Describes a baccalaureate nursing program's efforts to implement a community-focused curriculum to prepare nurses for a changed health-care system; reviews student program that includes mental health experience, health screening for preschoolers, and other clinical experiences.

Tagliareni, M. Elaine, and Joyce P. Murray. (1995). "Community-Focused Experiences in the ADN Curriculum." *Journal of Nursing Education* 34(8): 366-371.
Challenges traditional assumptions, values, and beliefs about associate's degree nursing education; based on the Community College–Nursing Home Partnership project.

Wilkinson, Judith M. (1996). "The C Word: A Curriculum for the Future." *Nursing and Health Care: Perspectives on Community* 17(2): 72-77.
Suggests that nursing education must be completely restructured to meet the health-care needs of the 21st century; describes a curriculum that would allow nurses to acquire appropriate depth and competence in the practice area of their choice.

General

Barber, Benjamin R., and Richard M. Battistoni. (1993). *Education for Democracy.* Dubuque, IA: Kendall/Hunt Publishing Co.
> Presents an anthology of readings on citizenship and social responsibility in a democracy, meant to provoke individual and group thought, discussion, and reflection.

Cha, Stephen, and Michael Rothman. (1993). *Service Matters: A Sourcebook for Community Service in Higher Education.* Denver, CO: Education Commission of the States.
> Compiles trends and statistics, national service initiatives, community service contacts, funding information, national organizations; includes more than 500 models and examples.

Coles, Robert. (1993). *The Call of Service: A Witness to Idealism.* New York, NY: Houghton Mifflin.
> Explores idealism in individuals and society, and community service as a means of realization; includes stories of individual involvement, achievement, and satisfaction, as well as cynicism, anger, and despair.

Council on Foundations. (1994). *A Grantmaker's Guide to National and Community Service.* Washington, DC: Council on Foundations.
> Provides information on national, state, and local foundations that award grants for national and community service efforts; includes program descriptions.

Education Commission of the States. (1994). *Federal Work-Study and Community Service: A Campus Compact Guide.* Denver, CO: Education Commission of the States.
> Reviews federal work-study legislation and its requirement of designated funds for community service work-study jobs; recommends strategies for implementation.

Fabiano, Patricia M. (1994). "From Personal Health Into Community Action: Another Step Forward in Peer Health Education." *Journal of American College Health* 43(3): 115-121.
> Examines how to translate health education's shift to a community orientation into practical, replicable steps forward in college peer health education; describes four assumptions in peer health education; explains a curriculum to reshape the philosophy of peer health education programs into a community- and service-oriented model.

Lappé, Frances Moore, and Paul Martin Du Bois. (1994). *The Quickening of America: Rebuilding Our Nation, Remaking Our Lives.* San Francisco, CA: Jossey-Bass.

> Chronicles individuals who are successfully tackling society's problems and challenges; addresses the skills needed to effect change and solve problems; includes reflective tasks and questions for the reader.

Pew Health Professions Commission. (1993). *Health Professions Education for the Future: Schools in Service to the Nation.* San Francisco. CA: Pew Health Professions Commission.

> Identifies characteristics of the emerging system, barriers to reform, and profession-specific recommendations for change.

Nursing Education

Eardley, Carla Jean. (1994). *Effective Tutoring for Nursing: A Guide for Peer Tutors.* Sacramento, CA: California Community Colleges.

> Lays the theoretical groundwork for understanding tutoring as a legitimate aspect of the larger field of learning assistance within a holistic framework.

Fairbrother, Patricia. (1996). "Recognition and Assessment of Teaching Quality." *Nurse Education Today* 16(1): 69-74.

> Identifies models for consideration of teacher quality and competence in nursing education; presents a range of evaluation criteria in preparation, delivery, innovation, communication, self-assessment, instructional management, peer recognition, professional memberships and service, publications, and grants and contracts secured.

Green, Anita J., and David G. Holloway. (1996). "Student Nurses' Experience of Experiential Teaching and Learning: Towards a Phenomenological Understanding." *Journal of Vocational Education and Training: The Vocational Aspect of Education* 48(1): 69-84.

> Relates interviews with nursing students who can define experiential learning, consider role playing the chief method, are aware of theory-practice issues, understand the importance of reflective practice, and view clinic supervision as an integral part of experiential learning.

Hall, Joanne M., and Patricia E. Stevens. (1995). "The Future of Graduate Education in Nursing: Scholarship, the Health of Communities, and Health Care Reform." *Journal of Professional Nursing* 11(6): 332-338.
Explains how graduate nursing education can be made more responsive to health-care needs in several ways: reflection on the roles of nurse practitioners and others, advocacy for vulnerable groups, expertise in community-based practice and research, understanding of the broader environmental context of health, and commitment to making a difference in public health.

Humbert, Pamela, and Lynn Barnett, eds. (1995). *Reaching Out: Associate Degree Nursing Programs at Work*. Washington, DC: American Association of Community Colleges.
Summarizes 27 community college nursing program models developed to bring more students into the nursing field and to help nursing programs meet community health needs.

Kelley, Barbara R. (1995). "Community-Based Research: A Tool for Community Empowerment and Student Learning." *Journal of Nursing Education* 34(8): 384-386.
Describes an urban university's experience using community-based research projects as a method of teaching nursing concepts and skills to beginning nursing students.

Lehna, Carlee, and Adrianne Byrne. (1995). "An Example of a Successful Collaboration Effort Between a Nurse Educator and a Hospice Clinical Nurse Specialist/Director." *Journal of Professional Nursing* 11(3): 175-182.
Suggests that collaboration between nursing education and nursing service recognizes the expertise of both educator and clinician; examines methods of promoting collaboration and explores its advantages and disadvantages.

Oesterle, Mary, and Darlene O'Callaghan. (1996). "The Changing Health Care Environment: Impact on Curriculum and Faculty." *Nursing and Health Care: Perspectives on Community* 17(2): 78-81.
Examines problems associated with the rapidly changing health-care system and resulting anxiety; suggests a shift in nursing education is necessary in order to provide competent primary health-care practitioners; describes an integrated primary health-care program.

Parker, David L., et al. (1995). "The Value of Critical Incident Analysis as an Educational Tool and Its Relationship to Experiential Learning." *Nurse Education Today* 15(2): 111-116.

> Reports how critical-incident analysis, combining actual experiences with structured reflection, can facilitate learning from clinical practice and development of interpersonal skills and self-awareness.

Rolfe, Andrew, et al. (1995). "A Dramatic Experience in Mental Health Nursing Education." *Nurse Education Today* 15(3): 224-227.

> Describes students in a mental health nursing program researching, writing, acting in, and evaluating a play about schizophrenia, demonstrating drama's effectiveness as a tool to develop sensitivity about health-care concerns.

Spier, Barbara Elliott. (1992). "Teaching Methodologies to Promote Positive Attitudes Toward the Elderly." *Nursing and Health Care* 13(10): 520-524.

> Recounts how attitudes change when nursing students are introduced to healthy elders in a community setting at long-term-care facilities.

Reflection

Goldsmith, Suzanne. (1995). *Journal Reflection: A Resource Guide for Community Service Leaders and Educators Engaged in Service Learning.* Washington, DC: American Alliance for Rights and Responsibilities.

> Relates the history and value of journals for service reflection, and details various types, formats, methods, and examples of journal reflection techniques.

Graham, Iain W. (1995). "Reflective Practice: Using the Action Learning Group Mechanism." *Nurse Education Today* 15(1): 28-32.

> Describes the action learning group, a strategy used in a nursing diploma/degree program to bridge the theory-practice gap; shows how techniques of reflective learning through group discussion allow students to become aware of the sources of their experience and beliefs, and to move toward accountability and responsibility.

Silcox, Harry C. (1993). *A How-to Guide to Reflection: Adding Cognitive Learning to Community Service Programs.* Philadelphia, PA: Brighton Press.
Details the need for reflection in service-learning, learning environments, reflective teaching methods, the reflection process, and research on reflection activities.

Stockhausen, Lynette. (1994). "The Clinical Learning Spiral: A Model to Develop Reflective Practitioners." *Nurse Education Today* 14(5): 363-371.
Addresses the clinical learning spiral, which incorporates reflective processes into undergraduate nursing education; entails successive cycles of four phases: preparative (briefing, planning), constructive (practice development), reflective (debriefing), and reconstructive (planning for change and commitment to action).

Service-Learning

American Association of Community Colleges. (1995). *Community Colleges and Service Learning.* Washington, DC: American Association of Community Colleges.
Describes in detail steps community colleges can take to implement service-learning.

————— . (1996). *Service Learning: A Community Strategy for HIV Prevention. A Teleconference of the Community College Satellite Network, Program Guide.* Washington, DC: American Association of Community Colleges.
Provides teleconference program and transcript of remarks; includes article on community college role in promoting community health, statistics on HIV infection and AIDS cases in the United States and worldwide, strategies for integrating service-learning and HIV prevention efforts, and suggested resources.

Ayers, George E., and David B. Ray, eds. (1996). *Service-Learning: Listening to Different Voices.* Fairfax, VA: United Negro College Fund.
Relates perspectives of educators from historically black colleges and universities regarding integrating service into academic curricula.

Berson, Judith S. (1994). "A Marriage Made in Heaven: Community Colleges and Service Learning." *Community College Journal* 64(6): 14-19.
Describes growth and relevance of service-learning in community colleges; discusses how to start service-learning programs.

Cauley, Katherine L., Cheryl A. Maurana, and Mary A. Clark. (1996). "Service-Learning for Health Professions Students in the Community: Matching Enthusiasm, Talent, and Time With Experience, Real Need, and Schedules." In *Expanding Boundaries: Serving and Learning*, edited by Jodi Raybuck, 54-57. Washington, DC: Corporation for National Service.
    Identifies opportunities, resources, and evaluation components for a multiinstitutional service-learning project.

Connolly, Charlene. (February 1996). "Rocky Chairland: Educating a Changing Health Care Workforce." Paper presented at the annual international conference of the National Community College Chair Academy, Phoenix, AZ.
    Details a community-based clinical practice incorporating service-learning as a structured part of the curriculum; recognizes the need to redefine the role of nursing and allied health practitioners at the associate's degree level, and transform curricula to meet the changing demands of health care.

Delve, Cecilia, Suzanne D. Mintz, and Greig M. Stewart. (1990). *Community Service as Values Education*. New Directions for Student Services, no. 50. San Francisco, CA: Jossey-Bass.
    Addresses how service-learning programs can foster students' moral development and sense of civic responsibility.

Galura, Joseph, Jeffrey Howard, Dave Waterhouse, and Randy Ross, eds. (1995). *Praxis III: Voices in Dialogue*. Ann Arbor, MI: OSCL Press.
    Describes service-learning courses and activities in detail; current thought and theory; and reflection by course alumni.

Galura, Joseph, Rachel Meiland, Randy Ross, Mary Jo Callan, and Rick Smith, eds. (1993). *Praxis II: Service-Learning Resources for University Students, Staff, and Faculty*. Ann Arbor, MI: OSCL Press.
    Discusses establishing a service-learning course and a faculty committee, advocating for and promoting service-learning on a university campus, pilot activities, and curricular and cocurricular projects.

Henry, Roger. (1995). *A Service Learning Center: A Practitioner's Workbook*. Cocoa, FL: Brevard Community College/Florida Campus Compact.
    Contains practical tips and suggestions for developing a service-learning program.

Howard, Jeffrey, ed. (1993). *Praxis I: A Faculty Casebook on Community Service-Learning*. Ann Arbor, MI: OSCL Press.
 Considers undergraduate and graduate course models of service-learning in a variety of disciplines; includes course structure, syllabi, outcomes, and assessment.

Jacoby, Barbara, and Associates. (1996). *Service-Learning in Higher Education: Concepts and Practices*. San Francisco, CA: Jossey-Bass.
 Outlines foundations and principles of viable service-learning programs; includes guidelines for program design and administration, types of service experiences, curricular integration, and institutionalization.

Kendall, Jane, ed. (1990). *Combining Service and Learning: A Resource Book for Community and Public Service*. 3 vol. Raleigh, NC: National Society for Internships and Experiential Education.
 Includes practical issues and ideas for programs and courses, curricular integration, recruitment, evaluation and assessment, legal issues, principles of good practice, theories, rationales, and research.

Kupiec, Tamar Y., ed. (1993). *Rethinking Tradition: Integrating Service With Academic Study on College Campuses*. Denver, CO: Education Commission of the States.
 Examines strategies and rationale for service-learning programs, service-learning as effective pedagogy, institutional development, program design; includes sample course syllabi.

Lepler, Marcia. (1996). "Service Learning Benefits Students, Communities." *NurseWeek* 9(4): 1, 22.
 Describes health-related service-learning programs at different institutions; recounts challenges and rewards of initiating service-learning.

Parsons, Michael H., and C. David Lisman, eds. (1996). *Promoting Community Renewal Through Civic Literacy and Service Learning*. New Directions for Community Colleges, no. 93. San Francisco, CA: Jossey-Bass.
 Portrays a critical role of community colleges in the 21st century as enhancing civic literacy through community-based programming and service-learning.

Robinson, Gail, and Lynn Barnett. (1996). *Service Learning and Community Colleges: Where We Are.* Washington, DC: American Association of Community Colleges.
Summarizes and analyzes service-learning data and trends on community college campuses.

Seidman, Anna, and Charles Tremper. (1994). *Legal Issues for Service-Learning Programs: A Community Service Brief.* Washington, DC: Nonprofit Risk Management Center.
Provides general guidance on legal liability, negligence, insurance, and risk management; suggests strategies to prevent legal problems; offers suggestions for adhering to pertinent laws and regulations.

Seifer, Sarena D., Sunita Mutha, and Kara Connors. (1996). "Service-Learning in Health Professions Education: Barriers, Facilitators, and Strategies for Success." In *Expanding Boundaries: Serving and Learning,* edited by Jodi Raybuck, 36-41. Washington, DC: Corporation for National Service.
Examines efforts to increase knowledge of service-learning in health professions education; describes a grant project's endeavors to identify barriers, facilitators, and success strategies at diverse institutions establishing service-learning.

Sigmon, Robert. (1994). *Linking Service With Learning.* Washington, DC: Council of Independent Colleges.
Relates service-learning background, typology, relationship identification, and suggestions for linking service with learning.

Troppe, Marie, ed. (1995). *Connecting Cognition and Action: Evaluation of Student Performance in Service Learning Courses.* Providence, RI: Education Commission of the States/Campus Compact.
Describes the importance and potential difficulty of evaluation in service-learning courses; offers evaluation methods and a model of the development of reflective judgment to assist faculty in assessing students' cognitive gains.

Westacott, Beverly M., and Carol R. Hegeman, eds. (1996). *Service Learning in Elder Care: A Resource Manual.* Albany, NY: Foundation for Long Term Care.
Describes elder-care project as a model for service-learning programs; includes case studies, curricular design, journal reflection, project evaluation, and mentoring information.

Appendix

List of Practitioners

Contributors to This Volume

Sharon P. Aadalen, PhD, RN
Associate Professor, Service Education Partnership
Mankato State University & Immanuel–St. Joseph's, Mayo Health System
School of Nursing, 27, College of Allied Health & Nursing
Mankato State University, Box 8400
Mankato, MN 56002-8400

Darlene A. Anderson, RN, DNSc
Assistant Professor
College of Nursing and Health
University of Cincinnati
Cincinnati, OH 45221-0038

Evelyn C. Atchison, RN, EdD
Program Director
School of Nursing
Northern Virginia Community College
8333 Little River Turnpike
Annandale, VA 22003-3706

Jean E. Bartels, PhD
Chair, Division of Nursing
Alverno College
P.O. Box 343922
3401 S. 39th Street
Milwaukee, WI 53234-3922

Leanne C. Busby, MSN, RNC, FNP
Assistant Professor of the Practice of Nursing
Family Nurse Practitioner Specialty Director
Project Director, W.K. Kellogg Grant
Vanderbilt University School of Nursing
Nashville, TN 37240-0008

Rev. Paul E. Carrier, SJ, PhD
University Chaplain and Director of Campus Ministry
Fairfield University
North Benson Road
Fairfield, CT 06430

Kate Cauley, PhD
Director, Center for Healthy Communities
Wright State University
3640 Col. Glenn Highway
Dayton, OH 45435

Elaine Cohen, EdD, RN
Private Consultant for Professional Practice, Outcome, and
    Performance Improvement
P.O. Box 10951
Fargo, ND 58106

Charlene Connolly, EdD
Division Chair
Health Technologies
Northern Virginia Community College
8333 Little River Turnpike
Annandale, VA 22003

Donna Miles Curry, RN, C, PhD
Associate Professor
College of Nursing & Health
Wright State University–Miami Valley
3640 Col. Glenn Highway
Dayton, OH 45435

L. Sue Davis, RN, PhD
Associate Professor
College of Nursing and Health
University of Cincinnati
Cincinnati, OH 45221-0038

Elizabeth Gardner, PhD
Professor
Psychology Department
Fairfield University
North Benson Road
Fairfield, CT 06430

Mary A. Glascoff, RN, MSN, EdD
Associate Professor and Director
Community Health Education
School of Health & Human Performance
East Carolina University
Greenville, NC 27858

Ruth Hanson, MS, RN
Internal Consultant
MeritCare Health System
720 Fourth Street, N
Fargo, ND 53122

Jean C. Hemphill, MSN, FNP, RNC
Assistant Professor
College of Nursing
East Tennessee State University
P.O. Box 70676
Johnson City, TN 37614-0676

Kimberley X. Hickok, RN, MS
Instructor
College of Nursing and Health
Wright State University–Miami Valley
3640 Col. Glenn Highway
Dayton, OH 45435

Mary Kay Hohenstein, RN, MEd
Instructional Dean
Health & Safety Division
South Central Technical College
1920 Lee Boulevard, Box 1920
North Mankato, MN 56002-1920

Mary I. Huntley, PhD, RN
Professor, Interim Associate Dean
Mankato State University & Immanuel–St. Joseph's, Mayo Health System
School of Nursing, 27, College of Allied Health & Nursing
Mankato State University, Box 8400
Mankato, MN 56002-8400

Susan Johnson, MS, RNC
Assistant Professor
Concordia College
901 S. 8th Street
Moorhead, MN 56562

Maryalice Jordan-Marsh, RN, PhD
Assistant Chair, Associate Professor
Department of Nursing
University of Southern California, Los Angeles
Center for the Health Professions
1540 Alcazar Street, CHP-222
Los Angeles, CA 90033

JoEllen Koerner, RN, PhD
Vice-President, Patient Services
Sioux Valley Hospital
1100 S. Euclid Avenue, Box 5039
Sioux Falls, SD 57105

Mary Kay Kohles, RN, MSW
Administration
Piedmont Hospital
1968 Peachtree Road, NW
Atlanta, GA 30309

Suzanne MacAvoy, RN, EdD
Professor
School of Nursing
Fairfield University
North Benson Road
Fairfield, CT 06430-7524

Carol L. Macnee, PhD, CS, RN
Associate Professor
College of Nursing
East Tennessee State University
P.O. Box 70676
Johnson City, TN 37614-0676

Annette J. McBeth, RN, MS, FAAN
Vice President
Immanuel–St. Joseph's, Mayo Health System
1025 Marsh Street, Box 8673
Mankato, MN 56002-8673

Margaret T. McNally, MA, RN
National Director
National Project Ladders in Nursing Careers (L.I.N.C.)
Greater New York Hospital Foundation, Inc.
555 W. 57th Street
New York, NY 10019

Lois Nelson, EdD, RN, CS
Chair and Professor
Concordia College
901 S. 8th Street
Moorhead, MN 56562

Jane S. Norbeck, RN, DNSc
Dean and Professor
School of Nursing
University of California-San Francisco
521 Parnassus Avenue, Box 0604
San Francisco, CA 94143-0604

Linda Norman, MSN, RN
Associate Dean for Academics
Assistant Professor
Vanderbilt University School of Nursing
Nashville, TN 37240-0008

Connie Peterson, MS, RN, CS
Assistant Professor
Concordia College
901 S. 8th Street
Moorhead, MN 56562

Evelyn D. Quigley, MN, RN
Vice President, Nurse Executive
MeritCare Health System
Fargo, ND 53122

Gail Robinson
Coordinator
Service Learning Clearinghouse
American Association of Community Colleges
One Dupont Circle, NW, Suite 410
Washington, DC 20036-1176
Internet: *grobinson@aacc.nche.edu*

Betty Sayers, MS
Management Consultant
RR1, Box 46A
Vergas, MN 56587

Nina P. Shah, MD
Centara Enterprises
Hampton, VA 23666

Cathy Taylor, MSN, RN
Assistant Professor of the Practice of Nursing
Vanderbilt University School of Nursing
Nashville, TN 37240-0008

Patricia A. Tumminia, MS, MEd
Professor
School of Nursing
Northern Virginia Community College
8333 Little River Turnpike
Annandale, VA 22003-3706

Deborah H. White, BA, MA
Director
Student Activities Center
East Tennessee State University
P.O. Box 70618
Johnson City, TN 37614-0618

Linda Workman, RN, PhD
Associate Professor
College of Nursing and Health
University of Cincinnati
Cincinnati, OH 45221-0038

Series Editor

Edward Zlotkowski is professor of English at Bentley College. Founding director of the Bentley Service-Learning Project, he has published and spoken on a wide variety of service-learning topics. Currently, he also is a senior associate on the AAHE Service-Learning Project at the American Association for Higher Education.

Directors of Service-Learning Projects Funded by the Corporation for National Service

*Evelyn C. Atchison

Shari Blumenthal, BS, MD Student '99
Student Director
HIPHOP
Robert Wood Johnson Medical School
675 Hoes Lane, Room N109
Piscataway, NJ 08854

---

*Also a contributor to this volume; for contact information, see pp. 181-187.

Michele Bush, MA
Director of Parenting Program
Gateway Community College
108 N. 40th Street
Phoenix, AZ 85034

*Kate Cauley

*Charlene Connolly

Kara Connors, BA
Program Coordinator
Health Professions Schools in Service to the Nation Program
UCSF Center for the Health Professions
1388 Sutter Street #805
San Francisco, CA 94109

Kathy Ferrer, BS, MD Student '99
Resource Manager
HIPHOP
Robert Wood Johnson Medical School
675 Hoes Lane, Room N109
Piscataway, NJ 08854

Rudy Filek, PhD
Director
West Virginia University
Robert C. Byrd Health Science Center
Office of Community and Continuing Education
Professional Education
P.O. Box 9009
Morgantown, WV 26506

Joanne Fussa, MS, RN, CSS
Coordinator, Learn & Serve: Higher Education
Primary Care
Center for Community Health, Education, Research, and Service (CCHERS)
Northeastern University
360 Huntington Avenue, 398 CP
Boston, MA 02115

---

*Also a contributor to this volume; for contact information, see pp. 181-187.

Carol Hegeman, MS
Co–Project Director
Foundation for Long Term Care
150 State Street
Albany, NY 12207

Kris Hermanns, BA, EdM
Associate Director
Swearer Center for Public Service
Box 1974
Brown University
Providence, RI 02912

Caryl Kramer, MS
Project H.E.A.L.T.H. Manager
West Virginia University
Robert C. Byrd Health Science Center
P.O. Box 9009
Morgantown, WV 26506

Yvonne LaRocca Lewis, EdD
Education Coordinator
AHEC Program
University of Arkansas for Medical Sciences
4301 W. Markham, Slot 559
Little Rock, AR 72205

*Suzanne MacAvoy

Jennifer Smith Sage, MPH
Program Coordinator
Everett Koop Institute at Dartmouth
7025 Strasenburgh
Hanover, NH 03755

---

*Also a contributor to this volume; for contact information, see pp. 181-187.

Sarena Seifer, MD
Director
Health Professions Schools in Service to the Nation Program
University of Washington
Box 351700
Seattle, WA 98195-1700

*Nina P. Shah

*Deborah H. White

---

*Also a contributor to this volume; for contact information, see pp. 181-187.